The Children's Vaccine Initiative

Achieving the Vision

Violaine S. Mitchell, Nalini M. Philipose,
and Jay P. Sanford, *Editors*

Committee on the Children's Vaccine Initiative:
Planning Alternative Strategies
Toward Full U.S. Participation

Division of International Health

INSTITUTE OF MEDICINE

NATIONAL ACADEMY PRESS
Washington, D.C. 1993

National Academy Press • 2101 Constitution Avenue, N. W. • Washington, D.C. 20418

NOTICE: The project that is the subject of this report was approved by the Governing Board of the National Research Council, whose members are drawn from the councils of the National Academy of Sciences, the National Academy of Engineering, and the Institute of Medicine. The members of the committee responsible for the report were chosen for their special competences and with regard for appropriate balance.

This report has been reviewed by a group other than the authors according to procedures approved by a Report Review Committee consisting of members of the National Academy of Sciences, the National Academy of Engineering, and the Institute of Medicine.

The Institute of Medicine was chartered in 1970 by the National Academy of Sciences to enlist distinguished members of the appropriate professions in the examination of policy matters pertaining to the health of the public. In this, the Institute acts under both the Academy's 1863 congressional charter responsibility to be an adviser to the federal government and its own initiative in identifying issues of medical care, research, and education.

Support for this project was provided by the Agency for International Development; the Department of Health and Human Services; the Pharmaceutical Manufacturers Association; the United Nations Development Program; and the World Health Organization, Children's Vaccine Initiative.

Library of Congress Catalog Card No. 93-84552
International Standard Book Number 0-309-04940-7

Additional copies of this report are available from:

National Academy Press
2101 Constitution Avenue, N.W.
Box 285
Washington, D.C. 20055

Call 800-624-6242 or 202-334-3313 (in the Washington Metropolitan Area)

B179

Printed in the United States of America

The serpent has been a symbol of long life, healing, and knowledge among almost all cultures and religions since the beginning of recorded history. The serpent adopted as a logotype by the Institute of Medicine is a relief carving from ancient Greece, now held by the Staatlichemuseen in Berlin.

COVER: Samantha Edington (age 4 years) provided the cover drawing for this report. Thanks are also due to Stefanie Hairston (5), Mira Kelada-Antoun (4), Stephanie Howson (6), Nadia Scott (4), and Anna Stoto (6).

COMMITTEE ON THE CHILDREN'S VACCINE INITIATIVE: PLANNING ALTERNATIVE STRATEGIES TOWARD FULL U.S. PARTICPATION

JAY P. SANFORD (*Chair*),* Dean Emeritus, Uniformed Services University of the Health Sciences, Dallas, Texas

MARY LOU CLEMENTS, Professor and Head, Division of Vaccine Sciences, Department of International Health, Johns Hopkins School of Hygiene and Public Health, Baltimore, Maryland

CIRO de QUADROS, Regional Advisor, Pan American Health Organization, Washington, D.C.

MICHAEL A. EPSTEIN, Partner, Weil, Gotshal & Manges, New York, New York

RONALD W. HANSEN, Associate Dean for Academic Affairs, William E. Simon Graduate School of Business Administration, University of Rochester, Rochester, New York

DONALD E. HILL, President, Don Hill & Associates, Silver Spring, Maryland

JOHN LLOYD HUCK (Retired), Former Chairman of the Board, Merck & Co., Inc., New Vernon, New Jersey

DAVID T. KARZON, Professor, Department of Pediatrics, and Department of Microbiology and Immunology, Vanderbilt University School of Medicine, Nashville, Tennessee

THOMAS D. KILEY, Attorney, Hillsborough, California

RICHARD T. MAHONEY, Vice President and Director, Technology Promotion, Program for Appropriate Technology in Health, Seattle, Washington

WENDY K. MARINER, Professor of Health Law, Boston University School of Public Health, Boston, Massachusetts

DAVID C. MOWERY, Associate Professor of Business and Public Policy, Walter A. Haas School of Business, University of California, Berkeley.

MARK NOVITCH, Vice Chairman of the Board, The Upjohn Company, Kalamazoo, Michigan

SURYANARAYAN RAMACHANDRAN, Immediate Past Secretary, Department of Biotechnology, New Delhi, India

ANTHONY ROBBINS, Professor of Public Health, Boston University School of Public Health, Boston, Massachusetts

JERALD C. SADOFF, Director, Division of Communicable Diseases and Immunology, Walter Reed Army Institute for Research, Washington, D.C.

---

* Member, Institute of Medicine

Preface

Vaccines are among the most cost-effective health interventions known. Indeed, the development and widespread use of vaccines in developed and developing countries have contributed greatly to the prevention of many devastating childhood diseases. Progress has been particularly impressive in the two decades since the establishment of the Expanded Program on Immunization under the leadership of the World Health Organization.

Unfortunately, a significant percentage of children, most in the poorest and most remote regions of the world, are not adequately immunized with existing vaccines. Underimmunization is also a problem in the United States, particularly among economically disadvantaged children living in rural and urban areas. Furthermore, no effective vaccines exist for a number of important infectious childhood illnesses. The Children's Vaccine Initiative was launched at the World Summit for Children in New York City in September 1990 to address these and other concerns related to childhood immunization.

This Institute of Medicine report, which addresses the central question, "How can the United States participate fully in the implementation of the Children's Vaccine Initiative?," provides important background information about the status of childhood immunization in this country and abroad, the available resources and infrastructure for producing vaccines, the supply of and demand for new and improved vaccines, the multistep process of vaccine research and development, and the dynamics of developing and manufacturing new and improved vaccines.

In developing our conclusions and recommendations, the Institute of

Medicine Committee on the Children's Vaccine Initiative has drawn on the expertise of individual committee members and has sought the participation and input of many individuals connected to the research, development, procurement, and supply of vaccines both domestically and internationally. The committee recognized early on in the study process that effective and efficient vaccine distribution and delivery systems are critical to ensuring the ultimate goal of disease prevention, but because this was not included in the charge to the committee, it is discussed only briefly in this report.

It is the conclusion of the Institute of Medicine Committee on the Children's Vaccine Initiative that the current system of vaccine research and development in the United States, which leads to the development of high-quality vaccine products for the domestic market, is unlikely to produce the majority of vaccines required by the Children's Vaccine Initiative. In addition, the committee believes that although the combined resources and expertise of the public and private sectors in the United States for the development and production of vaccines are both significant and impressive, they are not integrated and are not focused effectively on meeting public health goals. These conclusions led the committee to its major recommendation: the need for a National Vaccine Authority. The committee believes that a National Vaccine Authority, through a dynamic partnership between the public and private sectors, will offer the United States an extremely powerful tool to ensure the development of novel vaccines and vaccine technologies for use in immunization programs in the United States and around the world.

Publication of this report has been preceded by considerable national discussion about the desirability of having the U.S. government take a greater role in the purchase and distribution of vaccines recommended for use in U.S. children. The Institute of Medicine Committee on the Children's Vaccine Initiative did not study, and has not taken a position on an expanded federal purchase of vaccines. I believe I speak for the committee, however, when I say that certain sections of this report have relevance to the on-going discussion.

The committee forwards its recommendations having recognized that the curtailment of the burden of disease and death in the twenty-first century throughout the world, including within the United States, is another step toward the goal of a peaceful future for ourselves and our children.

Jay P. Sanford, *Chair*
Committee on the Children's Vaccine Initiative

Acknowledgments

Being asked to serve on, or in my instance to chair, an Institute of Medicine (IOM) committee is not a role that one assumes lightly. The Institute of Medicine does not address issues which are not of significant importance and social consequence, and the challenges of serving on an IOM committee are great and demanding. At the same time, one can be assured that one's colleagues will be dedicated to the task, expert in their fields, and collegial in their approach. One can also be confident that support by the IOM leadership and staff will be exceptional.

On behalf of the Institute of Medicine Committee on the Children's Vaccine Initiative, I would like to express our sincere appreciation to the numerous individuals and organizations who gave of their valuable time to provide information and advice to the committee. The committee would like to thank all the individuals who participated in the two working group sessions in June 1992 and who are listed in Appendix I. In addition, the committee would like to thank the following individuals who provided valuable information and advice to the committee: Kenneth Bart of the National Vaccine Program; Kenneth Bernard and Linda Vogel of the Office of International Health; Frank Cano and Jane Scott of Lederle-Praxis Biologicals; Glenna Crooks of Merck and Company, Inc.; George Curlin, Carole Heilman, John LaMontagne, Pamela McGinnis, Regina Rabinovich, and Dale Spriggs of the National Institute of Allergy and Infectious Diseases; Elaine Esber, M. Carolyn Hardegree, and Amy Scott of the U.S. Food and Drug Administration; Scott Halstead and Bruce Gellin of the Rockefeller Foundation; William Haussdorf, Pamela Johnson, Caryn Miller, and Michael White of the Agency for International Development; D. A. Henderson of the Department of Health and Human Services; Phyllis Freeman of the University of Massachusetts at Boston; Lance Gordon of ORAVAX; Sharon Mates of North American Vaccine; William Packer of Virus Research Institute; Ok Pannenborg of the World Bank; Philip K. Russell of Johns Hopkins University; Roy Widdus of the National Commission on AIDS; and Douglas Williams of Connaught Laboratories, Inc.

The committee gratefully acknowledges those who provided tables, graphs, funding data, and other information critical to the committee's deliberations: Janice Babcock of the Vaccine Project at the University of Massachusetts at Boston; Col. William Bancroft of the United States Army Medical Research and Development Command; Amie Batson, Peter Evans, and David Magrath of the World Health Organization; Matthew Berry and Geoffrey Evans of the Health Resources Services Administration; Timothy Brogan and Thomas Copmann at the Pharmaceutical Manufacturers Association; John Gilmartin and Terrel Hill of the United Nations Children's Fund; Tore Godal of the United Nations Development Program/World Health Organization/World Bank Special Program for Research and Training in Tropical Diseases; Akira Homma of the Pan American Health Organization; Major Robert Lipnick of the Department of the Army; Joseph McDade of the National Center for Infectious Diseases and Bill Nichols of the Division of Immunization at the Centers for Disease Control and Prevention; Robert Myers of the Michigan Department of Public Health; Lt. Col. Willis Reid of the Walter Reed Army Institute for Research; and Chester Robinson of the National Vaccine Program Office.

Finally, and in particular, the committee would like to express its appreciation of the Institute of Medicine staff who facilitated the work of this committee. We especially thank Violaine Mitchell, who assumed responsibility for the study midstream and was responsible for translating on-going discussions and debate into prose for further committee discussion; Nalini Philipose for her substantive and procedural contributions to the committee's work; and Dee Sutton, for her superb logistical support over the course of the study. The committee gratefully acknowledges the support and contribution of Stephanie R. Sagebiel who launched the study. Others within the IOM and National Academy of Sciences who were instrumental in seeing the project to completion were Michael Edington, Claudia Carl, and Betsy Turvene of the Reports and Information Office; Laura Baird, research librarian; Scott Jones, computer analyst; Sue Wyatt, financial associate; and Carolyn Hall, Dana Hotra, and Sharon Scott-Brown of the Division of International Health. Special thanks are due to Greg Pearson who edited and wrote sections of the report; Michael Hayes, editorial consultant; and Robert Crangle who facilitated the working group meetings in June 1992. The committee would also like to thank Kenneth I. Shine, IOM President; Enriqueta C. Bond, IOM Executive Officer; and Polly F. Harrison, Director of the Division of International Health, for their ongoing support of this study. The committee would also like to thank the study sponsors for their willingness to provide both support and input without attempting to influence the deliberations of the committee in any way.

Jay P. Sanford, *Chair*
Committee on the Children's Vaccine Initiative

Contents

APPENDIXES

Children represent the most vulnerable segment of every society . . .
they are our present and our future.

Declaration of New York, September 1990

The Children's
Vaccine Initiative

Achieving the Vision

1

Executive Summary

Vaccines are among the most affordable and effective health interventions available today. The development, introduction, and widespread use of vaccines in industrialized and developing countries have resulted in considerable progress against some of the most devastating of human diseases. Indeed, the world's only complete victory over an infectious agent resulted from a vaccine. Smallpox, which many believe caused more death and sickness than any other infectious illness, was eradicated from the world in the late 1970s. Public health officials in the Americas are now close to declaring victory over another infectious scourge: poliomyelitis.

Largely because of the success of the Expanded Program on Immunization (EPI; established in 1974, the EPI is administered by the World Health Organization and is supported by numerous national governments, international organizations, and private foundations), some 80 percent of the world's infants are adequately immunized against six important diseases: measles, tetanus, pertussis, diphtheria, tuberculosis, and polio. This is a remarkable achievement considering that just 20 years ago a scant 5 percent were so protected. Similarly, in the United States, cases of major infectious childhood diseases have dropped dramatically as vaccines have become a standard public health tool.

Despite tremendous progress in vaccinating children against some of the common infectious diseases, significant problems remain. A full 20 percent of the world's children, many in the poorest and most remote areas of the globe, are unvaccinated. And previously successful immunization efforts are showing signs of slipping, particularly in Africa south of the Sahara. More

1

than 2 million deaths and 5 million cases of disability still occur annually as a result of diseases (such as measles and *Haemophilus influenzae*) that are preventable by vaccination. In addition, a number of childhood diseases for which effective vaccines are not yet available, including malaria and acute diarrheal and respiratory infections, claim millions of lives annually.

The situation in the United States is also discouraging. Although almost all school-age children are well immunized, only about half of U.S. children under the age of 2 years have received the complete set of recommended immunizations, and the problem is particularly severe in inner-city areas and among indigent populations. The resurgence of measles in 1989 and 1990 was largely due to the failure of immunization programs to reach these groups. Most developed and many developing countries have achieved higher rates of immunization among their preschoolers than has the United States.

Vaccine delivery systems and schedules in the United States and the developing world are based on and restricted by existing vaccine-related technologies. Vaccines should be given early in life, when a child is most vulnerable to vaccine-preventable diseases. Most vaccines, however, require multiple administrations and, hence, multiple and costly contacts with the health-care system. And many vaccines require constant refrigeration. The complexity of vaccination schedules in the United States and much of the developing world exacerbates two categories of problems common to many immunization programs: high dropout rates and missed opportunities for vaccination.

THE CHILDREN'S VACCINE INITIATIVE

The last decade has brought significant advances in the science of vaccinology. Genetic engineering and other new vaccine technologies offer the promise of revolutionizing the ways that vaccines are made and simplifying the ways in which they are administered to children. It was the recognition of the role that science might play in developing new vaccines and improving currently available vaccines, and a perception that the translation of scientific advances into new vaccines needed by developing countries was lagging, that led to the Children's Vaccine Initiative (CVI).

The CVI is both a concept and an organization. The concept of the CVI was launched at the World Summit for Children in New York City in September 1990. The purpose of the CVI is to harness new technologies to advance the immunization of children. At the summit, it was proposed that the ideal CVI vaccine should be given as a single dose (preferably orally), effective when administered near birth, heat stable, contain multiple antigens, effective against diseases not currently targeted, and affordable. Making vaccines heat stable would eliminate the need for constant refrigeration, a critical limiting factor in the success and coverage of EPI programs in many countries. Combining more than one antigen into a single dose (as is now done with diphtheria and tetanus toxoids and pertussis vaccine [DTP], for instance) could dramatically reduce the number of vaccines and the costs required to immunize a child fully. Some characteristics of a CVI vaccine will be of public health value to the United States. Indeed, U.S. vaccine manufacturers are investing in research to develop new combination vaccines and simpler methods for administering vaccines. In addition, a new range of vaccines needs to be developed against diseases for which vaccines are not yet available.

The organization of the global CVI has evolved since the World Summit for Children. At the outset, the founders of the CVI (the Rockefeller Foundation, United Nations Development Program, United Nations Children's Fund, the World Bank, and the World Health Organization) recognized that no single agency or organization has the resources and capabilities to achieve the goals of the CVI. They recognized further that the CVI needed to involve many different entities to achieve the vision of the CVI. This recognition led to the formation of the CVI consultative group which is composed of representatives of national immunization programs, multilateral, governmental, and nongovernmental organizations, and commercial and public-sector vaccine manufacturers. The consultative group meets annually and provides an international forum for discussion of new CVI initiatives and for marshaling broad-based support for the CVI. The activities of the CVI itself are carried out through task forces and product development groups. The task forces examine strategic, logistic, and policy issues relevant to the industrial development and introduction of CVI vaccine products, including such areas as quality control, epidemiologic capability in developing countries, and global vaccine supply. The product development groups promote, facilitate, and manage projects leading to the development of vaccines and related products. The three current product development groups are focusing their efforts on a single-dose tetanus toxoid vaccine, a heat-stable oral polio vaccine, and an effective measles vaccine for administration earlier in life (see Chapter 2). The global CVI is headquartered at the World Health Organization in Geneva, Switzerland.

THE INSTITUTE OF MEDICINE REPORT

The Institute of Medicine (IOM) was asked by the two agencies responsible for formulating the U.S. response to the CVI–the U.S. Agency for International Development and the U.S. Public Health Service–to advise them on how to maximize U.S. private- and public-sector participation in the CVI.

The IOM, with financial support from the U.S. Agency for International Development, six U.S. Public Health Service entities (the Centers for Disease Control and Prevention, the U.S. Food and Drug Administration, Health Resources Services Administration, National Institute of Allergy and Infectious Diseases, National Vaccine Program Office, and the Office of International Health), the Pharmaceutical Manufacturers Association, the United Nations Development Program, and the World Health Organization, Children's Vaccine Initiative embarked in February 1992 on an 18-month study to:

• identify and explore major economic, legal, regulatory, policy, and other factors that influence, both negatively and positively, the development, production, introduction, and supply of vaccines; and
• recommend ways to enhance cooperation and participation among all relevant U.S. sectors in the realization of the CVI.

To conduct its work, the IOM convened an 18-member committee with a wide range of relevant expertise. The full committee met five times between February 1992 and February 1993. In addition, two multidisciplinary working groups comprising members of the IOM committee and other experts from concerned organizations met in June 1992. The committee members drew heavily on the proceedings of the working groups and their own experiences in identifying the major factors influencing U.S. participation in the CVI, reaching consensus on the relative importance of those factors, and recommending an approach to maximizing that participation.

COMMITTEE FINDINGS

Resources and Infrastructure

On the international front, national governments oversee immunization efforts in their respective countries. The Pan American Health Organization (PAHO), United Nations Development Program (UNDP), United Nations Children's Fund (UNICEF), World Health Organization (WHO), and the World Bank all contribute in various ways to efforts to develop vaccines and immunize the world's children. Furthermore, many nongovernmental organizations, such as the Rotary Foundation and Save the Children Fund, play a critical role in promoting protection from disease through immunization around the world. Although international commitment to universal childhood immunization is strong, the financial support for immunization activities provided by such agencies as WHO, UNICEF, and the Rotary Foundation has not kept pace with rising costs and increased demand for immunizations. In some cases, financial support for immunization activities has actually declined.

An extensive array of public agencies and private firms is involved in vaccine-related activities in the United States. Each year, the federal government spends hundreds of millions of dollars conducting research on new and improved vaccines, ensuring the safety of existing vaccines, purchasing and distributing vaccines to the states, and conducting educational and other outreach activities to encourage vaccine use.

The majority of basic research in the United States that leads to the development of new or improved vaccines is funded or conducted by the federal government, although a significant amount of basic research is conducted and funded by the private sector. Product-oriented research and development is conducted largely by established vaccine manufacturers and newly emerging biotechnology firms (development-stage firms). Over the last 10 years, development-stage firms have emerged as a new force in the area of applied vaccine research and early-stage product development. However, neither development-stage firms nor the federal agencies involved in vaccine research currently have the capability of manufacturing vaccines on a large scale. This is also true for Massachusetts and Michigan, the only two states that currently produce vaccines. The capacity to scale up and manufacture vaccines on a large scale rests almost entirely with a handful of commercial vaccine manufacturers.

Despite the substantial number and capabilities of U.S. government agencies, private firms, and other organizations involved in vaccine-related activities, and despite specific legislation mandating a national vaccine plan, there has been no overall strategy guiding research, production, procurement, and distribution of vaccines in the United States. As noted in a recent IOM report, ". . . the overall process of vaccine development, manufacturing, and use in the United States is fragmented. There is no direct connection between research and development on the one hand and use of vaccines on the other. The various decision makers do not work together; in fact, they respond to different pressures" (Institute of Medicine, 1992, p. 157). Similarly, and with specific regard to the CVI, the absence of a domestic strategy has, in the committee's judgment, impeded full U.S. participation in the CVI. U.S. government agencies interact with the global CVI virtually independently of each other.

Vaccine Demand and Supply

Demand

The potential size of the worldwide pediatric market is determined by two factors: the annual worldwide birth cohort (approximately 143 million live births per year) and the number of vaccines a child receives through adolescence.

Procurement of pediatric vaccines for the developing world tends to be highly concentrated, characterized by purchases of large numbers of doses by national governments or international agencies such as UNICEF or PAHO. UNICEF is the largest single buyer of vaccines for use in the developing world. In 1992, the fund purchased 850 million doses of childhood vaccines at a total cost of $65 million. The prices of vaccines procured by UNICEF are very low (it costs less than $1.00 to purchase vaccines to immunize a child against the six diseases mentioned above) and, until recently, have risen little more than the rate of inflation each year. Most companies that supply vaccines to UNICEF do so to utilize their excess capacity and charge prices that cover the marginal costs of production (costs of producing additional doses of vaccine in a fully capitalized and operational facility). Some major European suppliers of vaccine to UNICEF have indicated that the very low prices quoted to UNICEF are unlikely to be sustained into the future. Notably, no U.S. vaccine manufacturer has participated in the bidding or procurement process for UNICEF vaccines since 1982, the year in which a U.S. vaccine manufacturer was severely criticized in the U.S. Congress for selling vaccine at a lower price to developing countries than to the U.S. government for domestic needs. This continues to be a sensitive issue in the United States.

Compared with other pharmaceuticals, the demand for childhood vaccines in the United States is predictable, but limited. There are two major classes of buyers of childhood vaccines in the United States: the public sector (including the federal and state governments) and the network of private-sector physicians, health maintenance organizations, hospitals, pharmacies, and clinics across the country. Currently, a little more than half of all vaccines purchased are bought through 1-year contracts with federal or state funds at federally negotiated prices. In 1993 and as this report goes to press, President Clinton is proposing changes in the way that the federal government purchases and distributes pediatric vaccines.

Supply

Vaccines are manufactured in both developed and developing countries around the world by a range of producers, from vaccine divisions of large pharmaceutical companies to national institutes. Pasteur Mérieux Sérums et Vaccins (France) and SmithKline Beecham (United Kingdom) are the two largest suppliers of vaccines internationally and to UNICEF. There are also a number of national institutes in Europe and many developing countries that supply vaccines to meet their national needs. With a few exceptions, most national institutes have meager resources to conduct research on new and improved vaccines and have limited production capacities compared with those of commercial vaccine manufacturers. At this time, approximately 60 percent of the DTP used in developing countries is produced in the country in which it is used, and 80 percent of the children in the world are born in a country that produces at least one vaccine used in EPI. A number of countries are seeking to expand their capacity to manufacture additional vaccines to meet their domestic needs. There are, however, mounting concerns about the quality of vaccines produced in those countries that do not have a functional and independent regulatory authority.

Vaccine development and manufacture in the United States is an almost entirely commercial enterprise. Twenty years ago a dozen entities were making vaccines for U.S. children. Today, for a variety of reasons, nearly all childhood vaccines used in the United States are manufactured by four private companies. The supply of two vaccines is dependent on sole-source suppliers. The only two remaining public-sector vaccine manufacturers in the United States are the Michigan Department of Public Health and the Massachusetts Biologic Laboratories. Both entities manufacture vaccines to meet state needs, and both have active research and development programs with links to the private sector.

Innovation

The research and development of new and improved vaccines by commercial manufacturers exclusively for developing country markets is limited at best. The low prices quoted to UNICEF/PAHO cover the marginal costs of vaccine production, but they do not appear to provide sufficient market incentives for international vaccine companies to invest in research and development for exclusively developing-world vaccines.

Furthermore, despite a number of successful programs such as the WHO/UNDP Program for Vaccine Development or the UNDP/World Bank/WHO Special Program for Research and Training in Tropical Diseases, there is no significant international or multinational fund dedicated to the early stages of vaccine development and pilot testing of developing world vaccines.

New and improved vaccines that are developed and manufactured for industrialized-country markets do "trickle down" eventually (sometimes after many years) to some developing countries. By and large, however, the costs of new vaccines are beyond the means of most developing countries and such international buyers as UNICEF and PAHO. As a consequence, no new vaccines have been added to the UNICEF procurement system since its inception, despite recommendations by the World Health Organization that hepatitis B vaccine be included in national immunization programs.

The current vaccine development process in the United States, from basic research through to the production, distribution, and marketing of vaccine products, while poorly integrated, does lead to the development and production of new vaccines for the domestic market, primarily because vaccine manufacturers perceive there to be adequate returns on their investment. The current vaccine development system in the United States rarely leads to the development of vaccines intended for developing-country use, simply because such vaccines are perceived to be without sufficient returns on investment. In some cases, however, vaccines developed by or for the U.S. Department of Defense have been introduced into some developing countries on an *ad hoc* basis by commercial manufacturers.

Investing in New and Improved Vaccines

Private-sector manufacturers in the United States pursue the development of vaccines that both are technically feasible and have a market in industrialized countries. In some instances, a company may invest in the development of a technology with applications to the vaccine needs of both the United States and the developing world. For example, microencapsulation technology is under active investigation in the United States and abroad as a means of achieving a single-dose vaccine. In other instances, a company may be willing to undertake the development of a vaccine that is needed primarily in the developing world, if there are predictable markets of sufficient size and profitability. Such markets include members of the U.S. armed forces, U.S. travelers to developing nations, and wealthy segments of indigenous populations. In most instances, however, the development of new vaccines or improvements in existing vaccines targeted to populations in the developing world cannot be justified by commercial manufacturers. It is unrealistic to expect commercial vaccine manufacturers to bear the sole responsibility for the high-risk development and manufacture of vaccine products, such as those envisioned by the CVI, if the revenues received by manufacturers remain low.

Generally, a commercial manufacturer begins the process of vaccine development when scientific research has yielded promising results and when "proof of principle" (proof of principle is the point in research and development when the feasibility of a particular product or process is determined) has been established. The decision takes into account two critical factors: the technical feasibility and complexity of developing the vaccine and market considerations. Market considerations include the likelihood of a return on investment and the anticipated rate of return on investment, the availability of patent protection (and freedom from third-party claims of patent rights), and the potential costs of liability exposure.

Even if the technological feasibility of developing a vaccine product is established, commercial manufacturers may be unwilling to pursue development. The anticipated costs associated with research and development may be too high, patent issues may be too complex, the licensing process may present unacceptable obstacles, and the risks of liability may appear too great. The net effect of all of these concerns is increased risk. When the possibility of financial reward is perceived to be low, as is true under the present procurement system for most EPI vaccines, risk aversion will run high.

Stages of Vaccine Development

The process of vaccine development, manufacture, and use is often described as if it occurs in an ordered and linear fashion. In reality, taking a vaccine from the laboratory bench to the point at which a child is vaccinated is a difficult, complex, and iterative process. (The multiple stages of vaccine development are outlined in Chapter 6.)

The committee identified a number of impediments that hinder the ability of the U.S. public and private sectors to pursue the development and production of new and improved vaccines, including vaccines of potential use to the CVI.

Pilot Production

In the committee's judgment, a serious bottleneck to vaccine development is the relative scarcity of facilities that are used to manufacture pilot lots of vaccine according to FDA standards of current "Good Manufacturing Practices," an extensive body of regulations for manufacturing pharmaceuticals and biologics. Many of the vaccines currently under development, including those envisioned by the CVI, involve novel and experimental technologies and are directed against diseases for which there are no suitable animal models for evaluating vaccine efficacy. This new generation of vaccines will need to be evaluated early on and over time in carefully conducted human trials. Any vaccine used in safety and immunogenicity tests must be produced in a pilot production facility that meets "Good Laboratory Practices," and preferably current Good Manufacturing Practices. Although a number of private firms have the capability of producing pilot lots of vaccine on a small scale, few are able to produce pilot lots of vaccine that meet current Good Manufacturing Practices, and even fewer are able to scale up to large scale manufacture. Indeed, with the exception of a handful of publicly owned pilot production facilities operating in the United States, the capability of producing pilot lots of vaccine according to current Good Manufacturing Practices rests almost entirely with commercial vaccine manufacturers. For the most part, however, commercial pilot production facilities are oversubscribed and precedence is given to products with the highest commercial potential.

Clinical Trials

Clinical trials, especially phase III studies, are expensive (up to $20 million) and administratively and scientifically complex, and they must be carried out in locations with adequate health-care infrastructures. Although the vaccine evaluation units sponsored by the National Institute of Allergy and Infectious Diseases are a widely recognized and appreciated resource, many CVI vaccines will need to be tested in immunologically naive infants overseas, and this will pose additional challenges.

Scale-up and Large-Scale Manufacture

Manufacturers confront one of the most difficult, complex, time-consuming, and resource-intensive aspects of vaccine development when the decision is made to take a vaccine produced in small amounts in a pilot facility and scale up production to commercial levels. Licensing new and improved vaccine products also is complex and time-consuming, both for the manufacturer and for the U.S. Food and Drug Administration.

Technology Transfer

The international transfer of vaccine-related technology for CVI vaccines to developing countries raises several other potential problems. Many of the vaccines contemplated for use under the CVI will require production techniques and manufacturing facilities that are proprietary and, in some cases, more advanced than those that now exist outside of the United States and other developed nations.

A STRATEGY TO ENHANCE U.S. PARTICIPATION

Achieving the challenging vision of the CVI requires international commitment to the development and production of a new generation of vaccines. It is not only the health of those in the developing world that is at stake; the growing problem of immunization in the United States, especially among economically disadvantaged children, is a major concern.

Over the course of this study it has become increasingly clear to the committee that the current system of vaccine research, development, and manufacture in the United States that leads to the development of high-quality vaccines for the domestic market is not likely to produce the vast majority of vaccines needed for the CVI. This is primarily because most CVI vaccines targeted to developing countries lack the market potential of vaccines intended for the domestic market and do not provide adequate returns on investment in research and development.

At the same time, the committee recognizes that the scientific base for the development of new and improved vaccines in the United States is extensive and impressive and that new approaches and techniques to vaccine construction currently in research and development will revolutionize the ways that vaccines are made and delivered to children. The committee believes further, however, that U.S. public- and private-sector resources devoted to vaccine-related activities could be focused more effectively on meeting global public health needs.

The committee spent a great deal of time considering ways to maximize U.S. public- and private-sector participation in the global CVI and ensure that CVI vaccines are developed, manufactured, and made available to national EPI programs. The committee evaluated and rejected two major strategies for achieving full U.S. participation in the CVI (see Appendix D for a full discussion of strategies and options considered). The first strategy would have provided additional resources to federal agencies for CVI-related vaccine research and development. In addition, changes would have been made in the ways that the United States participates in the purchase and delivery of vaccines internationally. The second would have given the federal government the primary role in *all* phases of vaccine development, including large-scale vaccine manufacture and distribution. Both strategies were rejected because neither capitalized on the unique strengths and expertise of the newly emerging biotechnology firms and vaccine manufacturers in the United States, and neither strategy was thought likely to result in the timely development, production, and introduction of affordable CVI vaccines to developing countries.

The committee concurs with the findings of the recent Institute of Medicine report, *Emerging Infections* (Institute of Medicine, 1992), that the current process of vaccine innovation in the United States is fragmented and that an integrated process is required to ensure that needed vaccines that lack well-paying markets are developed and manufactured. The committee notes, however, that when stable, predictable, and long-term returns can be expected, commercial vaccine manufacturers have demonstrated their ability to manage and oversee the entire spectrum of activities required to take a vaccine from the point of proof of principle through to the point of production and distribution.

In the committee's view, the success of U.S. participation in the CVI will depend ultimately on effective cooperation and collaboration among government, universities, and most critically, the private sector, including both biotechnology firms and established vaccine manufacturers.

In the committee's judgment, the optimal way to maximize U.S. public- and private-sector participation in the global CVI and ensure that CVI vaccines are developed and manufactured for developing countries is to empower an entity to organize and manage an integrated process of CVI vaccine development and manufacture that not only builds and capitalizes on the strengths of the existing system but also has the capability and mandate to manage the vaccine development process from beginning to end. At this time, no federal entity, with the possible exception of the U.S. Department of Defense, has the capability of undertaking the breadth and range of activities required to ensure the integrated development, produc- tion, and procurement of CVI vaccines. In the committee's view, the development of new and improved vaccines for use in the industrialized countries and the developing world is unlikely to occur unless there is an entity that has the mandate to manage and oversee the process from start to finish.

Because the private sector alone cannot sustain the costs and risks associated with the development of many CVI vaccines,

the committee recommends that an entity, tentatively called the National Vaccine Authority (NVA), be organized to advance the development, production, and procurement of new and improved vaccines of limited commercial potential but of important public health need.

The NVA would be an organization within the U.S. government capable of reducing the risks and costs to industry associated with the development of CVI vaccines. The NVA would encourage private-sector firms, both biotechnology firms and commercial vaccine manufacturers, and academic and public-sector entities to develop products required for the CVI and would have an in-house capability to conduct applied research and development and manufacture pilot lots of vaccine.

The NVA would take full advantage of new and existing mechanisms for encouraging private-sector involvement in CVI-related research and development. Ideally, these might include guaranteed purchases of vaccine,[1] investment-tax credits for firms undertaking CVI-related activities, access to an NVA pilot production facility, financial and technical assistance with clinical trials, and provisions for limiting liability. In its agreements with private-sector partners, the NVA would retain the right to transfer the technology that it owns to developing countries, as appropriate. All such agreements would include strategies to ensure that whatever products result are affordable to markets in the developing world. The committee is well aware that the price of a vaccine cannot be determined at the outset of its development. However, the NVA could absorb many of the costs and risks associated with vaccine development.

It is likely that many vaccines would be developed exclusively by outside firms and entities with funding from the NVA. Other vaccines may require parallel tracks of development with collaboration between the private sector and the NVA. A few may require substantially more NVA involvement. The NVA would seek to transfer the responsibility for vaccine development to the private sector at every stage of the product development cycle, however. The NVA would support six broad areas of vaccine product development:

- vaccines used primarily in developing countries (e.g., shigella, cholera, salmonella, malaria, and dengue);
- improvements in existing vaccines which while not leading to a high market return would make them easier to distribute and administer or that would allow them to achieve immunity earlier in high-risk populations (e.g., heat-stable polio, single-dose controlled-release tetanus toxoid and other childhood vaccines, and a more immunogenic measles vaccine);
- development of simple, low-cost vaccine manufacturing technologies that could be easily transferred to vaccine manufacturers in developing countries;
- exploitation of vaccine technologies that are nonproprietary and therefore of little interest to commercial manufacturers who desire market exclusivity;
- adaptation and introduction of currently available vaccines (e.g., pneumococcal conjugates) and new vaccines, including combination vaccines, to developing countries; and

- vaccines for which there are small or limited markets or that are otherwise unprofitable.

The NVA would work with and make maximal use of existing resources at the U.S. Agency for International Development, the Centers for Disease Control and Prevention, the U.S. Department of Defense, the U.S. Food and Drug Administration, and the National Institutes of Health through interagency agreements for the conduct of basic research and clinical trials. Personnel from other government agencies and the private sector could be assigned to work at the NVA. Vaccines that are developed by the NVA and its partners would be licensed to commercial or public-sector manufacturers in the United States or to public-sector manufacturers in the developing world. The NVA would be an international resource and would work closely with the global CVI and multilateral organizations and institutions to ensure that vaccines developed by the NVA meet international needs.

The NVA would be a federal, or federally supported, entity. To be successful, it would have to have some characteristics not common to governmental organizations. The NVA would need to be able to purchase needed supplies and equipment quickly, renovate facilities, and build new research laboratories and pilot production facilities. It would need to have in-house regulatory expertise and staff experienced in negotiating issues related to intellectual property rights. In addition, some provisions must be made to limit the exposure of NVA's private-sector partners to claims of vaccine-related injury.

To be successful, the NVA must maintain a balance between its public health mission and its entrepreneurial activities. Having a board of directors drawn from the public health community, global CVI, multilateral organizations, U.S. government agencies, developing countries, academia, and the private sector (commercial manufacturers and biotechnology firms) would ensure that the NVA adheres to its mission.

The committee estimates that the up-front capital expense of establishing the NVA could range from $30 million to $75 million. The actual cost would depend on whether existing public-sector vaccine research and manufacturing capabilities are expanded or a new, freestanding unit is constructed and staffed. Each year, the NVA would require between $25 million and $45 million for grants, contracts, cooperative agreements, and other mechanisms to support its goals. Assuming annual operating costs and administrative services of $150,000–200,000 per person and a complement of 150–200 full-time staff, the annual operating budget would total $30 million. A total budget of $55 million to $75 million (extramural contracts and intramural operations) would be required. The NVA could also subsidize the vaccine prices paid by UNICEF and other agencies, and it could provide higher returns to private developers and manufacturers, where appropriate. Additional funds would need to be provided for this purpose.

The committee discussed where a new operational entity charged with the development of CVI products might be located (see Chapter 7 and Appendix D). A number of existing agencies might serve as home to the NVA, including the U.S. Agency for International Development, the Centers for Disease Control and Prevention, the Department of Defense, the U.S. Food and Drug Administration, the National Institutes of Health, and the National Vaccine Program Office. It is also possible, however, that the organization should be placed in a new, independent office.

Rather than recommend a specific site for the new entity, the committee developed a set of points to consider that it feels define the most important characteristics of any potential home for the NVA. These include the correlation of the existing agency's current mission to the mission of the NVA, the existing agency's intellectual and corporate culture and history, its track record in developing vaccines, and any potential conflicts of interest that may result from taking on the duties of the NVA. Although some agencies might meet more of the criteria than others, this fact alone does not necessarily identify the most appropriate location for the NVA. It is the committee's firm belief, however, that the NVA must be an operational entity with the capability, resources, and mandate to manage the entire spectrum of the vaccine development process from proof of principle to the procurement of required vaccines. At this time, no federal agency has the multidisciplinary capability required to manage the integrated development, production, and procurement of needed vaccines.

* * *

Vaccines are among the most cost-effective public health interventions available. Efforts to strengthen U.S and global vaccination efforts should be based on the research and development of new and improved vaccines. This committee forwards the recommendation for a National Vaccine Authority having recognized and struggled with the burden and discomfort that the proposal of creating a new entity brings.

An entity such as the NVA would fulfill a critical public health need and has the potential to protect children around the world while building on and strengthening public- and private-sector partnerships in the United States. The creation of an NVA will, for the first time, ensure the feasibility of a coherent program of development and production of CVI vaccines within the context and mandate of the 1986 legislation (P.L. 99-660) authorizing the National Vaccine Program and requesting the National Vaccine Plan.

The committee believes that the NVA, through a partnership between the public and private sectors, will offer the United States a new tool for ensuring the development of novel vaccines and vaccine technologies for use in immunization programs around the world and in the domestic public health arena.

The creation of an NVA-administered development and procurement program for CVI vaccines could greatly reduce the barriers to entry into vaccine production that many new biotechnology firms now face. By providing a market "springboard," this program could support the growth of U.S. biotechnology firms, potentially contributing to expansion in the sources of supply for other types of vaccine products, contributing to the growth of a U.S. biotechnology industry, and aiding in the bolstering of U.S. competitiveness in this important sector. In addition, U.S. participation in the CVI would constitute an extremely powerful, yet inexpensive contribution to developing countries. In the committee's view, the United States can and should play a decisive role in achieving the vision of the Children's Vaccine Initiative.

A Rationale for U.S. Participation in the CVI

Childhood immunization has led to remarkable declines in the incidence of sickness and death caused by vaccine-preventable diseases. This, in turn, has resulted in tremendous savings in costly and often long-term treatments.

Perhaps the greatest potential of immunization is the eradication of disease and the elimination of the need to vaccinate. The well-planned use of an effective vaccine made this goal a reality in the case of smallpox. By no longer having to vaccinate against this scourge, the United States alone is estimated to save $120 million per year. Hundreds of millions more are saved indirectly because of reductions in morbidity and mortality.

Polio is targeted as the next disease to be eradicated from the globe. Following an intensive vaccination campaign, there has not been a case of polio in the Americas since August 1991. Since the virus can be imported and spread from other parts of the world endemic for the disease, the United States and all countries in the Americas must be vigilant and continue to vaccinate against poliomyelitis. Vaccine-preventable diseases continue to occur in many nations of the world, often with a devastating impact on unimmunized segments of the population. There have been recent outbreaks of diphtheria in the Ukraine, measles in Somalia, and polio in Israel, to name but a few.

The United States has a long history of supporting immunization programs in other countries. Beyond the humanitarian underpinning of these efforts lies enlightened self-interest—it is in the United States' best interests to contribute to a world in which other nations are free from disease, disability, and their frequent correlate, poverty.

Vaccine-preventable diseases are an economic drain on developing countries. Developing countries that are able to sustain a healthy and productive work force—through effective disease prevention activities, including immunization—are more likely to become vibrant and full partners in the international community. As such, they not only are able to support a domestic economy but also provide a market for the goods and services of other countries. Currently, according to the U.S. Department of Commerce, almost a third of all U.S. exports go to the developing world, and this amount is likely to increase in the years to come.

Critics argue that vaccinating more of the world's children will lead inevitably to more people, more poverty, and a greater drain on finite natural resources. It is true that over 80 percent of births occur in so-

Continues

called developing countries. Yet it has been demonstrated in many different settings that enhancing child survival leads to a decline, not an increase, in the birth rate. Families that can be assured that a child will survive are more likely to have fewer children.

Although most of the attention of the global Children's Vaccine Initiative (CVI) is focused on the needs of children in the developing world, most of the vaccines and technologies that will be developed are of importance to children in the United States. Vaccines that are effective in a single dose—either through enhanced immunogenicity or the use of technologies such as sustained release—will be of great value in the United States. The reemergence of a number of dangerous infectious diseases poses new challenges. New and more effective vaccines against pneumonias, measles, meningitis, and tuberculosis are needed in both the United States and developing countries.

By supporting global efforts at health promotion, an initiative like the CVI clearly has indirect economic benefits for the United States. There are direct benefits too. A significant number of scientists working on new and improved vaccines are based in the United States—in universities, in government laboratories, in biotechnology firms, and in vaccine manufacturing companies. Many of the world's most innovative vaccine manufacturers are U.S.-based. Thus, supporting the CVI will, to a large extent, support the U.S. scientific and biotechnology enterprise and can advance the development of vaccines for the public health needs in the United States. And investing in and supporting vaccine development and immunization programs will have guaranteed and lasting dividends to us all.

NOTE

1. This proposed mechanism resembles the defense procurement process. During the 1950s and 1960s, DOD procurement played a critical role in launching a number of small, start-up firms in the semiconductor and computer electronics industries. By providing large purchase orders to producers of semiconductors that met its specifications, the DOD enabled fledgling producers to expand their revenues. These producers would have found it more difficult to enter commercial markets for their devices, because these markets are associated with much higher marketing and distribution costs. Analyses of the semiconductor and other high-technology industries have argued that the effects of DOD procurement were more important than the effects of DOD research and development contracts on the entry and growth of new firms.

REFERENCE

Institute of Medicine. 1992. Emerging Infections. Washington, D.C.: National Academy Press.

2

Why a Children's Vaccine Initiative?

PROGRESS TOWARD
UNIVERSAL CHILDHOOD IMMUNIZATION

Vaccines are among the most affordable and effective health interventions available today. The development, introduction, and widespread use of vaccines in industrialized and developing countries have resulted in considerable progress against some of the most devastating infections of humankind. Indeed, the world's only complete victory over an infectious agent resulted from a vaccine. Smallpox, which many believe caused more death and sickness than any other infectious disease, was eradicated from the world in the late 1970s following a well-planned and highly effective vaccination campaign. Public health officials in the Americas are now close to achieving a similar victory over another infectious scourge: poliomyelitis.

One of the largest and most successful efforts to date to capitalize on the tremendous potential of vaccines is the Expanded Program on Immunization (EPI). The EPI, which is headquartered at the World Health Organization (WHO) and supported by numerous individual governments, non-governmental organizations, and bilateral and multilateral agencies, was established in 1974. Its aim was to build on the success of WHO's Smallpox Eradication Program and to assist national immunization programs in the developing world. To advance the goal of universal childhood immunization, the EPI supports national governments in their efforts to implement effective vaccine delivery programs.

Among the greatest hurdles faced by the EPI during its first years of operation was starting national immunization programs where none had existed before (Robbins, 1991). Political commitment to the goals of the EPI had to be secured from more than 90 countries. Immunization personnel had to be trained, systems had to be established to deliver and monitor immunization efforts, and adequate national and international resources had to be put in place to support the massive undertaking.

Armed with vaccines against just six diseases—diphtheria, pertussis, tetanus, tuberculosis, polio, and measles—the EPI has made remarkable strides toward achieving universal childhood immunization. By the end of 1991, an estimated 80 percent of the world's infants were reported to be vaccinated with BCG (bacillus Calmette-Guérin, the antigen used to vaccinate individuals against tuberculosis), measles vaccine, diphtheria and tetanus toxoids and pertussis vaccine (DTP), and oral polio vaccine (OPV) (Pan American Health Organization, 1993; UNICEF, 1992). Each year, EPI-sponsored immunization programs prevent some 2.9 million deaths from measles, neonatal tetanus, and pertussis as well as 440,000 cases of polio worldwide (Kim-Farley et al., 1992; Pan American Health Organization, 1993; World Health Organization, 1992).

This great achievement stands in sharp contrast to the situation in the mid-1970s, when less than 5 percent of the developing world's children were adequately immunized and when nearly 5 million children died each year from vaccine-preventable diseases (UNICEF, 1989).

Limits of the Expanded Program on Immunization

Despite tremendous progress during the 1980s toward the goal of universal immunization coverage, there is concern that the success of the six-vaccine EPI effort cannot continue indefinitely (Claquin, 1989, 1990; Poore et al., 1993; REACH Project, 1990; Robbins and Freeman, 1988; Rosenthal, 1990). Each year, a new and larger cohort of children at risk for vaccine-preventable diseases must be immunized. Some 20 percent of the world's children, many in the poorest and most remote areas of the world, have yet to be reached at all by national immunization programs (Pan American Health Organization, 1993). Indeed, more than 2 million deaths and 5 million cases of disability still occur as a result of diseases that are preventable by vaccination (Pan American Health Organization, 1993; Ransome-Kuti, 1991).

It is also worth noting that the six existing vaccines offered through EPI offset only a fraction of the burden of infectious diseases affecting children in developing countries (Figure 2-1). For example, acute diarrhea causes 3 million to 5 million deaths annually and accounts for at least one third of

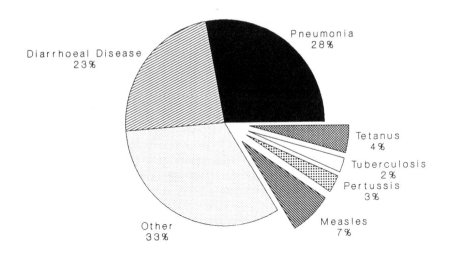

FIGURE 2-1 Under-five deaths by cause, developing countries, 1990. Cut slices: Vaccine-preventable diseases. SOURCE: State of the World's Children, 1993.

the deaths in children under age 5 years. Acute respiratory infections kill more than 2 million people every year (Ransome-Kuti, 1991), and an estimated 1 million to 2 million people, most of them children, die from malaria each year (Institute of Medicine, 1991). Vaccines for these three sets of conditions are in various stages of development but are not yet available for use.

These concerns, coupled with the recognition that genetic engineering and new vaccine technologies could permit the development of a new generation of childhood vaccines and that the translation of these scientific advances to vaccines needed by developing countries was lagging, led to the establishment of the Children's Vaccine Initiative (CVI).

THE CHILDREN'S VACCINE INITIATIVE

The CVI is both a concept and an organization. The initial focus of the CVI, launched after the World Summit for Children in New York City in September 1990, was to accelerate efforts to develop vaccines that could enhance the performance of EPI (World Health Organization/Children's Vaccine Initiative, 1991a, 1992). A number of specific, desirable features of future children's vaccines were proposed (see the box "What Is the Children's Vaccine Initiative?"). Vaccines incorporating some or all of these characteristics offered the potential for protecting more of the world's children against a larger number of diseases at a lower cost per child or per disease prevented (Robbins, 1991). As secondary, longer-term objectives, it was hoped that the CVI could facilitate efforts to ensure an adequate supply of vaccines for children in the developing world and simplify the complex logistics of vaccine delivery.

Over time, the mission and goals of the CVI have matured. In particular, those involved in the initiative recognized that vaccine development, production, and delivery cannot be considered independently–they are intimately linked. Underlying this shift in thinking has been the realization that the manufacture of vaccines cannot be assured without taking into account the prospective development of new and improved vaccines. Vaccine development, in turn, cannot be successful without taking into account such issues as demand, intellectual property rights, production capabilities, and technology transfer.

The organization of the global CVI has also changed since the World Summit for Children. The founders of the CVI (the Rockefeller Foundation, United Nations Development Program [UNDP], United Nations Children's Fund [UNICEF], the World Bank, and the WHO) recognized at the outset that no single agency or organization has the resources and capabilities to achieve the goals of the CVI. They recognized further that the CVI needed to involve many different entities to achieve the vision of the CVI. This recognition led to the formation of the CVI consultative group, which is composed of representatives of national immunization programs, multilateral agencies, nongovernmental organizations, development-stage firms, commercial vaccine manufacturers, public-sector vaccine manufacturers, and national development assistance agencies. The consultative group, which meets annually, provides an international forum for discussion of new CVI initiatives and for marshaling broad-based support for the CVI.

The activities of the CVI are carried out primarily through product development groups and task forces. CVI task forces examine strategic, logistic, and policy issues relevant to the industrial development and introduction of CVI vaccine products. Task forces focused on the following topics have been established to date: priority setting and strategic planning, relations with vaccine development collaborators, situation analysis of the global vaccine supply, assessment of national vaccine regulatory capabilities and needs, and strengthening national epidemiological capacities to ensure the best use of vaccines. A new task force on the management of DTP combinations for the developing world has been proposed as a means to plan, coordinate, and implement a global effort to ensure the development and supply of quality DTP combination vaccines to developing countries. However, these activities are likely to be beyond the capabilities of a single task force and will need to be implemented through other means as well

---

What Is the Children's Vaccine Initiative?

The Children's Vaccine Initiative (CVI), is an international effort to harness new technologies to advance the immunization of children. At the World Summit for Children in New York City in September 1990, world leaders called for an acceleration of the application of current science to the development of new and improved childhood vaccines. Preceding the summit, world vaccine experts proposed a number of desirable features for future children's vaccines. They are that the vaccines be:

- single dose,
- administered near birth,
- combined in novel ways,
- heat stable,
- effective against diseases for which vaccines are unavailable, and
- affordable.

The goals of the CVI have matured. Those involved in the initiative have come to recognize that vaccine development is intimately linked to issues of vaccine production and supply. These issues deserve equal consideration. Underlying this shift in thinking is the realization that the manufacture of vaccines cannot be assured without taking into account the prospective development of new vaccines. Development, in turn, cannot be successful without taking into account such issues as local production, intellectual property rights, technology transfer, and collaboration with the private sector.

The Children's Vaccine Initiative, which is headquartered at the World Health Organization in Geneva, Switzerland, is cosponsored by five organizations: the United Nations International Children's Fund, the United Nations Development Program, the Rockefeller Foundation, the World Bank, and the World Health Organization.

(Philip K. Russell, Johns Hopkins University, personal communication, 1993).

The CVI product development groups promote, facilitate, and manage projects that lead to the development of vaccines and related products. The three current product development groups are focusing their efforts on a single-dose tetanus toxoid vaccine, a heat-stable oral polio vaccine, and an effective measles vaccine for administration earlier in life. The heat-stable oral polio vaccine and single-dose tetanus toxoid product development groups, which were formed in late 1991, are working with a few academic and industrial partners and have identified some promising techniques. The measles product development group became operational in March 1993. Other product development groups will be established as needs and priorities are identified and objectives set.

The success of the CVI depends on the cooperation of vaccine manufacturers, governments, and multinational organizations, such as UNICEF and the Pan American Health Organization, which supply vaccines to much of the developing world. Effective cooperation will allow vaccine developers to create new and improved vaccines of use to suppliers, and it will help the suppliers make long-term plans that take into account the vaccines of the future.

Characteristics of CVI Vaccines

The long-term goal of the CVI is to develop a means of immunizing children at birth against all important disease threats with a single proce-dure. World vaccine experts who met before the World Summit for Children agreed upon six desirable features of future childhood vaccines. They should be single dose, administered near birth, combined in novel ways, heat stable, effective against additional diseases, and affordable. A vaccine that has some or all of these characteristics has the potential to save money, thereby allowing more money to be spent on reaching the 20 percent of children in the world who are currently unprotected (Robbins, 1991; World Health Organization/Children's Vaccine Initiative, 1991b). Some vaccines developed by the CVI will be targeted exclusively for the populations of developing countries (e.g., shigella, malaria, and dengue); others, such as combination vaccines made up of existing and improved vaccines (e.g., DTP-hepatitis B vaccine combinations), are needed by the populations of both industrialized and developing countries.

Vaccines Should Be Single Dose

Protecting a child against the six basic childhood diseases currently requires adherence to a complicated vaccination schedule (see Appendix G). The WHO immunization schedule recommends that children receive single doses each of BCG and OPV at birth and then three doses of DTP and OPV each at ages 6, 10, and 14 weeks. Measles vaccine is administered at age 9 months. The complexity of the vaccination schedule contributes to and exacerbates two categories of problems common to many immunization programs: high dropout rates and missed opportunities for vaccination (de Quadros et al., 1992). Whether because of the lack of information, difficulty getting to the health clinic, or inappropriate clinic hours, families may not take their children for necessary and additional booster shots, and thus drop out of the vaccination program. In other instances, health-care workers may not check whether a child requires any immunizations during a visit to a health clinic for reasons other than vaccination. In either case, children may not receive important vaccinations. Efforts to track and completely immunize every child are labor and resource intensive (de Quadros et al., 1992). Reducing the number of required vaccine doses to protect a child fully, and hence the number of contacts with the health-care system, would reduce costs and lead to enhanced coverage against disease.

Vaccines Should Be Administered Near Birth

Some currently available vaccines, for example, measles vaccine, are not immunogenic in very young children because of interference from maternal antibody. Yet by the time the vaccine is administered to an older infant, the child may already have been exposed to or contracted the disease. A vaccine that could be administered near birth would have a substantial impact on the incidence of some vaccine-preventable diseases in young children.

Vaccines Should Be Combined in Novel Ways

The discomfort of injections and the effort required to bring children to health clinics discourages many necessary visits. Combination vaccines would reduce the number of required contacts with the health-care system by protecting against more diseases in a single administration. Integrating combination vaccines into the existing vaccine schedule could be done at minimal cost—the cost of the vaccine itself—since investments in vaccine delivery systems have already been made. Major efforts are under way around the globe to develop combination vaccines by using DTP as the base to which additional antigens can be attached (Chapter 4).

There are a number of novel vaccine delivery systems in various stages of research and development that have the potential to ease vaccine administration; some such systems may even obviate the need for booster doses, needles, and syringes. Sustained-release vaccines, for example, would release immunogenic antigens over time, thereby foregoing the need for subsequent doses. Increased widespread use of oral vaccines could eliminate patient concerns about the discomfort associated with injections. Not only would clinic visits be more tolerable to patients but the costs and risks of using syringes and other equipment would also be reduced. Children could receive many vaccinations at one time, painlessly (Robbins, 1991).

Vaccines Should Be Heat Stable

Without refrigeration, vaccines have a limited usable shelf-life, and refrigeration and maintenance of the "cold chain" have been critical limiting factors of EPI in many countries (de Quadros et al., 1992; Pan American Health Organization, 1993). An immunization program can extend only as far as the cold chain permits. By extension, an immunization program is only as effective as its cold chain.

The cold chain is expensive and difficult to operate and maintain (de Quadros et al., 1992; Pan American Health Organization, 1993), demanding refrigeration at every stop along the route from the central manufacturing facility to the point at which a child is vaccinated (Table 2-1). The public health costs when the cold chain fails are much higher, however. In such cases, children may receive ineffective vaccines. The result may be a serious erosion of public confidence in the immunization program as children become sick with the very disease against which they were vaccinated. It has been estimated that the costs associated with enhancing or extending the cold chain approach half of the total costs of immunization programs (de Quadros et al., 1992).

Increasing the heat stability of vaccine could extend the immunization efforts while at the same time reducing vaccine wastage and the cost of refrigeration. Heat-stable vaccines could be carried by health-care workers to areas previously inaccessible because of the limitations of the cold chain. The number of vaccine failures resulting from a temperature-related loss of potency could be markedly reduced (de Quadros et al., 1992).

Vaccines Should Be Effective Against Additional Diseases

The current set of vaccines offered through EPI has inherent limits. Six antigens can control only six diseases. Many other vaccine-preventable diseases are managed by less effective and often more costly methods of

TABLE 2-1 Maximum Storage Times and Temperatures for Selected Vaccines at Various Points from the Central Store to the Health Center

Vaccine	Central Store (up to 8 months)	Regional Health Post (up to 3 months)	Health Center (up to 1 month)	Transport (up to 1 week)
Measles				
Yellow fever	−15 to −25°C			
Oral polio				
DTP				
Tetanus toxoid		0 to 8°C		
Diphtheria and tetanus toxoids				
BCG				

NOTE: DTP and tetanus toxoid freeze below -3°C; storage times are recommended maximum figures.

SOURCE: Robbins (1988–1989).

prevention or treatment.

There are many diseases against which vaccines may be a useful preventive tool, including malaria, which kills more than 1 million children each year, pneumococcal disease in children, and rotavirus. In 1986, in response to a request from the National Institute of Allergy and Infectious Diseases, the Institute of Medicine evaluated the costs and potential benefits of over 20 new or improved vaccines of importance to the developing world (Institute of Medicine, 1986a,b). The development costs, in 1985 dollars, were estimated to range between $10 million and $50 million per vaccine. Since that time, the UNDP/WHO Program for Vaccine Development has undertaken similar priority-setting exercises, as is the CVI itself (see Chapter 6) (World Health Organization, 1991; World Health Organization/Children's Vaccine Initiative, 1992, 1993).

In the last 10 years, WHO has sought to encourage researchers to study the health challenges facing developing countries. The UNDP/WHO Program for Vaccine Development and the UNDP/World Bank/WHO Special Program for Research and Development in Tropical Diseases, for example, were both created to bring laboratory investigators face-to-face with the problems encountered in the field. The Program for Vaccine Development is primarily a research-stimulating and research-supporting effort. The participants in the program, almost exclusively research scientists, have worked to bring vaccine research to "proof of principle," the point at which product development can begin. Proof of principle is the point at which the most intensive CVI efforts are needed. However, certain technologies that are important in early vaccine development, such as technologies to achieve a single dose or heat stability, will also be a focus of the CVI.

It was once hoped that if the public sector identified the needs and funded basic research, private industry would develop technically feasible vaccines (Institute of Medicine, 1992; World Health Organization/Children's Vaccine Initiative, 1991a). However, as discussed in subsequent chapters of this report, this has not yet happened; the barriers and impediments to the development of vaccines for the industrialized and the developing world are complex and variable.

Vaccines Should Be Affordable

The affordability of vaccines is of critical importance to EPI programs (Kim Farley et al., 1992; Robbins and Freeman, 1988). Vaccine costs currently represent only about 10 percent of the overall expense of administering EPI (Figure 2-2), but a very large percentage of the foreign exchange input into national immunization programs (John Gilmartin,

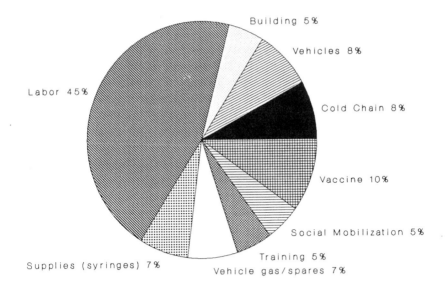

FIGURE 2-2 Estimated distribution of Expanded Program on Immunization delivery costs. Note: This breakdown is an average global estimate. Actual costs vary considerably from country to country. Supervision costs range from 3 to 5 percent of labor costs. SOURCE: Amie Batson, World Health Organization/Expanded Program on Immunization, 1992.

UNICEF, personal communication, 1993). It now costs EPI an estimated $15 to immunize a child living in a developing country; the cost of the vaccine amounts to less than $1 (Kim-Farley et al., 1992). Not included in this calculation are investments in capital infrastructure, such as the health centers where children are vaccinated.

Studies conducted at the start of the EPI program found that it cost approximately $5.00 to immunize one child, with the cost of vaccine amounting to $0.50 (Robbins, 1991). The increased cost of immunizing a child in 1993 is not due to rising vaccine and material costs alone (supplies, transportation, cold chain equipment, and facilities), the latter of which have actually decreased (Robbins, 1991); rather, it suggests that the children who were most easily vaccinated were immunized first, increasing the per-child cost of vaccinating the remaining children (Robbins, 1991).

If past experience is any indication, the prices of new and improved vaccines on the international market fall over time. Since it was first available 10 years ago, for example, hepatitis B vaccine has dropped to less than one one-hundredth of the original price (Mahoney, 1990; Maynard, 1989). Advances in technology and competition seem likely to bring down the price of the *Haemophilus influenzae* type b vaccine (Hib) as well. The introduction of Hib and hepatitis B vaccine could be the first major additions to EPI since its inception. One critical area of concern to CVI and EPI is how to ensure that new vaccines are affordable to developing countries when they first appear on the market. Adding new and improved vaccines to the EPI, whether such vaccines are purchased from international suppliers or produced locally, will inevitably increase the costs to EPI. For this reason, the committee's recommended strategy, outlined in Chapter 7, includes provisions that could change the current system for the development of affordable vaccines and the procurement of vaccines, subsidizing the prices paid by UNICEF and other agencies, and providing higher returns to private developers and manufacturers, where appropriate.

Concerns About the CVI

Some critics of the CVI approach to vaccine innovation argue that resources would be better spent improving means of delivering existing vaccines to currently underserved populations rather than developing new and more sophisticated vaccines. Others have cautioned that the prices of new vaccines may prohibit their use in developing countries (Kim-Farley et al., 1992) or lead to a reduction in existing coverage under EPI. At the same time, the sustainability of even the existing EPI is being called into question (Claquin, 1989, 1990; Poore et al., 1993; REACH Project, 1990). Many developing countries rely on outside support for their immunization programs and are unlikely to be able to sustain these efforts in the future without a continued infusion of outside resources (Claquin, 1989, 1990; REACH Project, 1990; Rosenthal, 1990); thus, expanding the program depends upon persuading donor organizations to provide more funding for global vaccine procurement (an unlikely strategy in the light of scarce resources and competing priorities) or reducing the costs of immunization. The costs of EPI can be lowered primarily in two ways: reducing the number of contacts required to protect a child and distributing vaccines that are easier to administer and that are less dependent on refrigeration. CVI is seeking to tackle both of these areas.

There is a range of complicated and practical impediments to introducing new and technologically complex vaccines into EPI. Integrating new vaccines into the EPI will require some retraining of over 100,000 health-care workers—a Herculean task. Furthermore, countries that currently make some vaccines for their populations may not have access to, or in some cases the capability to manufacture, novel vaccines that employ complex technologies. It is feared that the capability and know-how to manufacture new vaccines will be tightly held by only a few vaccine manufacturers. Indeed, without an effort to ensure that all children have access to new and improved-quality vaccines, children in industrialized countries will have access to the new combination vaccines, while children in developing countries will remain dependent on single-antigen vaccines and will not be protected from additional important diseases (e.g., malaria and acute respiratory infections).

RELEVANCE OF THE CVI TO U.S. IMMUNIZATION EFFORTS

Status of Immunization Efforts in the United States

The use of childhood vaccines in the United States has caused the number of cases of diphtheria, an acute bacterial infection, to fall from nearly 6,000 in 1950 to 3 or 4 a year currently (U.S. Department of Health and Human Services, 1992). Cases of pertussis (whooping cough), another illness caused by a bacterium, have dropped from over 120,000 in 1950 to 4,500 in 1990 (U.S. Department of Health and Human Services, 1992). The incidence of measles, a viral illness, has fallen off dramatically in the last 30 years, despite a major increase in 1990 (U.S. Department of Health and Human Services, 1992). Similar dramatic reductions in disease incidence have been reported for mumps, polio, rubella (German measles), and most recently, *Haemophilus influenzae* type b (U.S. Department of Health and Human Services, 1992).

As a counterpoint to this record of achievement against many infectious diseases is the disappointing reality that a significant proportion of children under the age of 5 years, the most vulnerable age group for vaccine-preventable diseases, are not fully vaccinated (Cutts et al., 1992a,b; National Vaccine Advisory Committee, 1991; Peter, 1992; Schlenker et al., 1992). For example, in 1985, the last year for which national data are available, only 55 percent of U.S. preschoolers received three or more doses of polio vaccine; just 65 percent were fully vaccinated with DTP (U.S. Department of Health and Human Services, 1992). Vaccine coverage rises sharply after age 5 years–to over 95 percent–since all states require proof of adequate immunization prior to enrollment in school (Cutts et al., 1992a,b; Hinman, 1991; Plotkin and Plotkin, 1988).

The Centers for Disease Control and Prevention (CDC), in conjunction with state and local health departments, recently completed retrospective assessments of vaccine coverage in 20 U.S. cities (Centers for Disease Control and Prevention, 1992a). Data from nine cities indicate that although 90 percent of children had one vaccination before their first birthday and although most children began their vaccinations on schedule, fewer than half of the children surveyed were fully immunized by age 2 years

(Centers for Disease Control and Prevention, 1992b). Another recent survey of 51 immunization projects nationwide indicated that the overall immunization levels of children under 2 years of age were low, with 16 projects reporting immunization levels below 50 percent (Centers for Disease Control and Prevention, 1992b).

Other industrialized and developing countries have been able to achieve higher rates of immunization. For example, in 1990, over 97 percent of Swedish, Danish, and Swiss children were reported to be fully immunized against polio by 1 year of age, as were over 95 percent of 1-year-olds in Pakistan, Costa Rica, and Mexico (Liu and Rosenbaum, 1992; UNICEF, 1992, 1993).

To improve immunization levels in preschool-age children, CDC embarked on an Infant Immunization Initiative with state and local health departments in 1991 (Centers for Disease Control and Prevention, 1992). The goal of the initiative is to develop novel strategies in vaccine delivery (Centers for Disease Control and Prevention, 1992a; Freeman et al., 1993). Although the U.S. Public Health Service has set a goal for the year 2000 of ensuring 90 percent immunization coverage for preschoolers (U.S. Department of Health and Human Services, 1992), given the current rates of vaccination, few believe that this goal will be attained. In fact, immunization levels among children under age 5 years for many diseases have actually declined since the late 1970s (Liu and Rosenbaum, 1992; U.S. Department of Health and Human Services, 1992).

From a public health perspective, this trend is alarming. A fundamental principle of disease control by vaccination is that enough people must be immunized to maintain so-called herd immunity. When vaccine coverage drops below a certain level, local outbreaks and, potentially, epidemics are possible. The resurgence of measles during the late 1980s and early 1990s is an example of what can happen when vaccination is carried out incompletely and vaccination rates are low (National Vaccine Advisory Committee, 1991; Schlenker et al., 1992). The number of reported cases of measles in 1990 (27,786) was the highest since 1977 and was nearly 20-fold more than was documented in 1983, the year the fewest number of cases was reported. About half of the reported cases in 1990 were among preschool-age children; among vaccine-eligible preschoolers, nearly 80 percent were unvaccinated (Cutts et al., 1992a; National Vaccine Advisory Committee, 1991).

A Role for the CVI in the United States

Despite the relatively plentiful supply of childhood vaccines in the United States, many children do not undergo the complete series of recommended immunizations on time. Although it was not the mandate of this committee

Despite the relatively plentiful supply of childhood vaccines in the United States, many children do not undergo the complete series of recommended immunizations on time. Although it was not the mandate of this committee to address this particular concern, many of the barriers that prevent children in the United States from receiving the full benefit of vaccines are similar to those in other parts of the world. These include missed vaccination opportunities, deficiencies in the health-care delivery system (most acutely in the public sector), inadequate access to health care, and lack of public awareness of required immunizations (National Vaccine Advisory Committee, 1991; Peter, 1992; Schulte et al., 1991; Szilagyi et al., 1993).

As in other parts of the world, the vaccination schedule for U.S. children, developed by the CDC's Advisory Committee on Immunization Practices, is complex (see Appendix G). Children living in the United States are required to receive more vaccines than children living in countries taking part in EPI (ten versus six). Achieving complete immunization in the United States entails a minimum of five visits to the doctor before age 2 years and additional visits at ages 4–6 years, 14–16 years, and every 10 years thereafter. The actual number of visits to a health-care provider is considerably higher, since many parents and pediatricians prefer to spread the number of immunizations out rather than give three or four shots in one sitting.

The sheer number of vaccines and contacts with the health-care system required to fully protect a child has led U.S. vaccine manufacturers to pursue the development of combination vaccines (see Chapter 4). Many of these products will be as useful to EPI as they are to the public health goals of the United States. In many respects, then, the United States and countries served by the EPI are facing a similar set of problems, and there is potential for overlap in the solutions being considered. Therefore, the vaccine development efforts of U.S. firms have relevance and are of vital interest to the international CVI.

REFERENCES

Brenzel L. Costs of EPI: 1990. A Review of Cost and Cost-Effectiveness Studies (1979-1989). REACH Project. Arlington, Virginia: John Snow, Inc.

Centers for Disease Control and Prevention. 1992. Retrospective survey results of immunization status of children at second birthday by immunization project: school year 1991/1992. Letter from Walter A. Orenstein, December 15.

Centers for Disease Control and Prevention. 1992b. Retrospective assessment of vaccination coverage among school-aged children–selected U.S. cities, 1991. Morbidity and Mortality Weekly Report 41(6):103–107.

Claquin P. 1989. Sustainability of EPI: Utopia or Survival? REACH Project. June. Arlington, Virginia: John Snow, Inc.

Claquin P. 1990. Overview of Issues in the Sustainability of EPI. REACH Project. October. Arlington, Virginia: John Snow, Inc.

Cutts FT, Orenstein WA, Bernier RH. 1992a. Causes of low preschool immunization coverage in the United States. Annual Review of Public Health 13:385–398.

Cutts FT, Zell ER, Mason D, Bernier RH, Dini EF, Orenstein WA. 1992b. Monitoring progress towards U.S. preschool immunization goals. Journal of the American Medical Association 267:1952–1955.

Day LM. 1990. Toward Ensuring the Financial Sustainability of EPI. REACH Project. October. Arlington, Virginia: John Snow, Inc.

de Quadros CA, Carrasco P, Olive JM. 1992. Desired field performance characteristics of new improved vaccines for the developing world. Paper presented at the NIAID Conference on Vaccines and Public Health: Assessing Technologies and Global Policies for the Children's Vaccine Initiative, November 5–6, 1992, Bethesda, Maryland.

Freeman P, Johnson K, Babcock J. 1993. A health challenge for the states: Achieving full benefit of childhood immunization. Occasional Paper. February. The John W. McCormack Institute of Public Affairs, University of Massachusetts at Boston.

Hinman AR. 1991. What will it take to fully protect all American children with vaccines? American Journal of Disease Control 145:559–562.

Institute of Medicine. 1991. Malaria: Obstacles and Opportunities. Washington, D.C.: National Academy Press.

Institute of Medicine. 1986a. New Vaccine Development: Establishing Priorities. Volume I. Diseases of Importance in the United States. Washington, D.C.: National Academy Press.

Institute of Medicine. 1986b. New Vaccine Development: Establishing Priorities. Volume II. Diseases of Importance in the Developing World. Washington, D.C.: National Academy Press.

Institute of Medicine. 1992. Emerging Infections. Washington, D.C.: National Academy Press.

Kim-Farley R and The Expanded Programme on Immunization Team. 1992. Global immunization. Annual Review of Public Health 13:223–237.

Johnson KA. 1987. Who's Watching Our Children's Health? December. Washington, D.C.: Children's Defense Fund.

Liu JT, Rosenbaum S. 1992. Medicaid and Childhood Immunizations: A National Study. Children's Defense Fund. January. Washington, D.C.

Mahoney RT. 1990. Cost of plasma-derived hepatitis B vaccine production. Vaccine 8:397–402.

Maynard JE. 1989. Global control of hepatitis B through vaccination: Role of hepatitis B vaccine in the Expanded Programme on Immunization. Reviews of Infectious Diseases 11(Suppl. 3):S574–S578.

National Vaccine Advisory Committee. 1991. The measles epidemic. Journal of the American Medical Association 226:1547–1552.

National Vaccine Advisory Committee. 1992. Access to Childhood Immunizations: Recommendations and Strategies for Action. April. Rockville, Maryland.

Pan American Health Organization. 1992. Progress in the worldwide polio eradication effort. EPI Newsletter 14(6):1–2.

Pan American Health Organization. 1993. Global EPI progress reviewed. EPI Newsletter 15(1):6.

Peter G. 1992. Childhood immunizations. New England Journal of Medicine 327:1795–1800.

Plotkin SL, Plotkin SA. 1988. A short history of vaccines. Vaccines, Plotkin SA and Mortimer EA, eds. Philadelphia: W.B. Saunders Company.

Poore P, Cutts F, Seaman J. 1993. Universal childhood immunization: Is it sustainable? Lancet 341:58.

Ramachandran S Russell PK. 1992. Draft. A new technologic synthesis: The Children's Vaccine Initiative. Paper presented at the NIAID Conference on Vaccines and Public Health: Assessing Technologies and Global Policies for the Children's Vaccine Initiative, November 5–6, 1992, Bethesda, Maryland.

Ransome-Kuti O. 1991. Introductory remarks. Meeting of the Consultative Group, Children's Vaccine Initiative. December 16–17, 1991. World Health Organization, Geneva.

REACH Project. 1990. Immunization Sustainability Study. April. Arlington, Virginia: John Snow, Inc.

Robbins T. 1988–1989. Prospectus from WHO, EPI Technical Series: The Cold Chain Product Information Sheets, No. 1. Geneva: World Health Organization.

Robbins T. 1991. The Children's Vaccine Initiative: A prospectus. September. Boston University School of Public Health. Unpublished.

Robbins T Freeman P. 1988. Obstacles to developing vaccines for the Third World. Scientific American. November. 126-133.

Rosenthal GR. 1990. The Economic Burden of Sustainable EPI Implications for Donor Policy. REACH Project. February. Arlington, Virginia: John Snow, Inc.

Schlenker TL, Bain C, Baughman AL, Hadler SC. 1992. Measles herd immunity. Journal of the American Medical Association 267:823–826.

Schulte JM, Bown GR, Zetzman MR, Schwartz B, Green G, Haley CE, Anderson RJ. 1991. Changing immunization referral patterns among pediatricians and family practice physicians, Dallas County, Texas, 1988. Pediatrics 87:204–207.

Szilagyi PG, Rodewald LE, Humiston SG, Raubertas RF, Cove LA, Doane CB, Lind PH, Tobin MS, Roghmann KJ, Hall CB. 1993. Missed opportunities for childhood vaccinations in office practices and the effect on vaccination status. Pediatrics 91(1):1–7.

UNICEF. 1989. The State of the World's Children. Oxford: Oxford University Press.

UNICEF. 1992. The State of the World's Children. Oxford: Oxford University Press.

UNICEF. 1993. The State of the World's Children. Oxford: Oxford University Press.

U.S. Congress, House. 1986. Childhood Immunizations. A report prepared by the Subcommittee on Health and the Environment, Committee on Energy and Commerce. September. Washington, D.C.

U.S. Department of Health and Human Services. 1992. Health United States 1991. May. Hyattsville, Maryland.

World Health Organization. 1991. Programme for Vaccine Development: A WHO/UNDP Partnership. December. Geneva.

World Health Organization. 1992. EPI for the 1990s. Geneva.

World Health Organization/Children's Vaccine Initiative. 1991a. Meeting of the Consultative Group. Geneva.

World Health Organization/Children's Vaccine Initiative. 1991b. Why a Consultative Group on the Children's Vaccine Initiative and Why Now? December. Geneva.

World Health Organization/Children's Vaccine Initiative. 1992. Meeting of the Consultative Group. Geneva.

World Health Organization/Children's Vaccine Initiative. 1993. Task Force on Priority Setting and Strategic Planning. Geneva.

3

Resources and Infrastructure

Global resources and infrastructures for the development, production, and supply of vaccines are large, and their full documentation is beyond the scope of this study. In this chapter, the committee seeks to give the reader a perspective on the number and variety of participants in immunization activities, both in the United States and internationally.

RESOURCES IN THE UNITED STATES

The United States supports a large number of public agencies and programs involved in vaccine-related activities (National Vaccine Advisory Committee, 1992). Each year, the federal government spends hundreds of millions of dollars to conduct research for new and improved vaccines, ensure the safety of existing vaccines, purchase and distribute vaccines to the states, and conduct educational and other outreach activities to encourage vaccine use. The U.S. government does not currently produce vaccines on a large scale, that is the province of private industry. However, both Massachusetts and Michigan manufacture vaccines for their respective populations.

The bulk of federally supported vaccine research and development is funded by the National Institutes of Health (NIH), primarily through the National Institute of Allergy and Infectious Diseases (NIAID); the Centers for Disease Control and Prevention (CDC); the U.S. Agency for International Development (AID); the U.S. Department of Defense (DOD), largely through the Departments of the Army and Navy; and the U.S. Food and Drug Administration (FDA). DOD and CDC purchase vaccines at federally negotiated contract prices and distribute them to the military and civilian sectors, respectively. Regulatory oversight and licensure are performed by FDA's Center for Biologics Evaluation and Research (CBER). Demonstration projects, field testing, and postmarketing surveillance for vaccines are conducted or funded by AID, CDC, and FDA. The National Vaccine Program (NVP), which is part of the Office of the Assistant Secretary for Health of the U.S. Department of Health and Human Services, is authorized to coordinate and provide direction to the nation's various vaccine-related efforts; this mandate is carried out under the guidance of the National Vaccine Advisory Committee, which is composed of representatives of government agencies, public health experts, private industry, and citizens groups.

U.S. Federal Agencies and Programs

U.S. Agency for International Development

The U.S. Agency for International Development participates in a wide range of immunization-related activities. On the domestic front, AID representatives participate as liaison members to the NVP's National Vaccine Advisory Committee (NVAC). In addition, they sit on the U.S. Department of Health and Human Services' NVP Interagency Group, whose membership comprises senior scientific and policy officials from AID, CDC, DOD, FDA, NIH, and NVP and is charged with overseeing implementation of the NVP.

AID's vaccine-related initiatives are international in scope. The bulk of AID resources supports national EPI programs and is provided through bilateral agreements. Since 1986, AID has committed an estimated $246 million for immunization programs and vaccine-related research to more than 60 countries (U.S. Agency for International Development, 1992). In 1991, AID allocated over $15 million for the development and testing of vaccines (Institute of Medicine, 1991; U.S. Agency for International Development, 1992). AID funds also support the development, testing, and introduction of diagnostics and immunization-related technologies intended to simplify vaccine administration and improve the "cold chain" (the system needed to keep vaccines refrigerated from manufacture to administration). AID has provided extensive support to strengthen the developing world's capacity for vaccine testing and delivery and for disease surveillance. The agency funds the development of epidemiological and research capacity in developing countries and provides grant support for epidemiology and field testing.

In 1992, AID initiated a set of specific responses to the international Children's Vaccine Initiative (CVI) (U.S. Agency for International Development, 1992). These included a grant program to support research on CVI-related topics conducted jointly by scientists from the United States and less-developed countries. AID also has provided funding for the Vaccine Independence Initiative, sponsored by the United Nations Children's Fund (see International Resources, below).

Center for Biologics Evaluation and Research,
U.S. Food and Drug Administration

The Center for Biologics Evaluation and Research at FDA is responsible for the scientific review of license applications for new biologics, including vaccines. CBER examines new biologics submitted by vaccine manufacturers for safety and efficacy, as well as process consistency and regulatory compliance. In addition to its role in licensing vaccines and facilities that manufacture vaccines, CBER has active laboratory research and postmarketing surveillance programs that complement and support its regulatory activities. CBER also works closely with scientific committees at the World Health Organization (WHO) and is working toward greater international harmonization of vaccine standards.

In fiscal year 1992, CBER had a total of 641.3 full-time equivalent positions (FTEs) (Center for Biologics Evaluation and Research, Office of Management, 1993). The operating budget was $24,365,000, and the payroll, including salaries and benefits, was $36 million (Center for Biologics Evaluation and Research, Office of Management, 1993). The number of FDA FTEs engaged in vaccine activities was 223, and FDA allocated over $27 million to CBER's vaccine work (Center for Biologics and Evaluation Research, Office of Management, 1993), $14.9 million of which was directed toward research and development for children's vaccines (World Health Organization/Children's Vaccine Initiative, 1993). CBER has also received support from the National Vaccine Program Office (NVPO) (U.S. Department of Health and Human Services, 1992). In fiscal year 1991, the NVPO provided eight FTEs and almost $1.9 million to FDA, permitting the agency to enhance the development of a safer pertussis vaccine, establish a computer tracking system to analyze the lot-specific relationships of reports of adverse events, and work on projects associated with the CVI (Kessler, 1992; U.S. Department of Health and Human Services, 1992).

FDA representatives actively participate on WHO technical and expert committees, which review and set international technical standards for biologics. FDA staff also sit on several CVI task forces and product development groups. In addition, the FDA is actively involved in the International Conference on Harmonization, which includes the European Community, Japan, and the United States and addresses global standardization. For the most part, the International Conference on Harmonization has thus far addressed technical requirements for drugs. The FDA conducts bilateral activities with the European Community, Mexico, Canada, and the United Kingdom; these activities consist primarily of information sharing and discussion of broad regulatory policy issues. Finally, the FDA carries out bilateral activities with a number of countries, including Egypt, India, and Russia–activities that are largely funded by AID.

Centers for Disease Control and Prevention

The Centers for Disease Control and Prevention is charged with protecting the health of U.S. citizens. CDC's vaccine-related activities are carried out by its Division of Immunization. CDC purchases 50–60 percent of all public-sector doses of vaccine recommended for general use in the United States. Every year, CDC negotiates consolidated federal contracts with manufacturers for routinely recommended childhood vaccines. These public-sector rates are substantially lower than those charged the private sector (see Chapter 4). CDC makes grants to the states to purchase the vaccines at the contract price. In fiscal year 1992, CDC funded the purchase of $154 million worth of vaccines. An additional $18.7 million was awarded to the states to support immunization program operations, and another $12.8 million was targeted at efforts to manage follow-on activities related to the measles outbreak of 1989–1990 (Centers for Disease Control and Prevention, Division of Immunization, 1992).

In addition to the purchase of vaccines, CDC helps states and localities determine their immunization needs and plan and implement immunization programs. Among other tasks, states must distribute and administer vaccines, develop and maintain systems that can be used to detect adverse events associated with vaccination, conduct disease surveillance, assess immunization levels, and provide professional educational materials about the importance of vaccination. CDC also has developed the national vaccine stockpile, currently having a 26-week reserve of most childhood vaccines, to manage any short-term interruption in supply. The agency, along with the FDA, monitors the Vaccine Adverse Events Reporting System, a surveillance network which receives reports of the adverse events that occur within specified time frames following vaccination.

Although CDC's efforts are focused primarily on U.S. health needs, the agency does participate in immunization-related activities on a global level.

TABLE 3-1 NCID Expenditures in Research, Development, and
Clinical Trials for Selected Vaccines in Fiscal Year 1992

Vaccine	Research and Development ($)	Clinical Trials ($)
Dengue	282,000	
Haemophilus influenzae type b	25,000	
Hepatitis B		368,000
Malaria	143,000	
Measles	25,000	
Meningitis	130,000	140,000
Pertussis	247,000	
Pneumococcus	272,000	
Polio	154,000	130,000
Streptococcus (group a)		32,000
Streptococcus (group b)	25,000	
Venezuelan equine encephalitis	20,000	
Total	1,459,000	

SOURCE: Joseph McDade, Office of the Director, National Center for Infectious Diseases, Atlanta, Georgia, May 1993.

The majority of research and training in the area of infectious diseases supported by the CDC is conducted by the National Center for Infectious Diseases (NCID) (Table 3-1). Although CDC does not sustain overseas laboratories, it does support overseas field stations that conduct research and training in infectious diseases as collaborative activities with the host country. The agency has approximately 50 employees based in foreign countries, many of whom are working on infectious disease activities. In fiscal year 1990, the agency responded to 25 international public health emergencies, 10 of which were related to infectious disease outbreaks (Institute of Medicine, 1992).

CDC's Epidemic Intelligence Service provides training and field experience in epidemiology to health professionals. Epidemic Intelligence Service officers are assigned to CDC headquarters, CDC's domestic field stations, state and local health departments, or other federal agencies to carry out epidemiological research and investigations. This program is a model for the joint CDC/WHO Field Epidemiology Training Program. The programs are funded by the host country and countries with epidemiologists who can assist in the development and implementation of disease control and prevention programs (Institute of Medicine, 1992).

TABLE 3-2   Amount of Vaccine Distributed to Army Installations by the Defense Logistics Agency in Calendar Year 1991

Vaccine	No. of Doses Purchased	Price/Dose ($)	Total Cost ($)
Measles-mumps-rubella	251,000	18.66	4,700,454
Diphtheria and tetanus toxoids and pertussis	253,950	8.15	2,069,693
Polio (oral)	474,100	2.44	1,156,804
Meningococcal	196,100	3.83	751,063
Plague	374,514	0.79	295,866
Rabies	8,576	49.79	426,999
Typhoid (parenteral)	31,220	0.55	17,171
Yellow fever	227,560	3.29	748,672
Hepatitis B	19,122	23.85	456,060
Adenovirus (type 7)	120,800	0.65	78,520
Adenovirus (type 4)	108,000	0.65	70,590
Total	2,066,442		10,769,892

SOURCE: Robert J. Lipnick, Disease Surveillance Officer, U.S. Army Medical Material Agency, Frederick Maryland, October 6, 1992.

U.S. Department of Defense

The U.S. Department of Defense is both a purchaser of vaccines and an active vaccine research and production entity. In calendar year 1991, DOD's procurement arm, the Defense Logistics Agency, bought some $10.7 million worth of vaccine at government-negotiated prices (Table 3-2). The total spent by DOD on vaccines is thought to be on the order of two to three times this amount, however, since many DOD units buy vaccine directly from the manufacturer. The vaccines, including at least three intended for use in the developing world (plague, typhoid, and yellow fever), are distributed to various Army installations by the Defense Logistics Agency.

In fiscal year 1992, DOD spent a total of $76.7 million on vaccine-related research, $42 million of which supported work on vaccines against human immunodeficiency virus (HIV), the virus that causes AIDS (Table 3-3). As the lead agency for infectious disease research, the Army provides the U.S. Naval Medical Research Institute $10 million annually. However, DOD vaccine research is conducted mostly by the Division of Communicable Disease and Immunology at the Walter Reed Army Institute of Research, which employs approximately 220 people and spends roughly $15 million annually. Vaccine research and development is also conducted at the U.S. Army Institute of Infectious Diseases (USAMRIID) at Fort Detrick,

TABLE 3-3   Infectious Disease Vaccine Research by the U.S. Defense Department in Fiscal Year 1992

Area of Vaccine Research	Fiscal Year Cost (in millions of $)
Viral diseases	14.1
Bacterial diseases	8.1
Malaria vaccine research	7.9
Nonenteric bacteria	4.6
HIV/AIDS	42.0
Total	76.7

SOURCE: COL William Bancroft, Director, Military Diseases Hazards Research Program, U.S. Army Medical Research and Development Command, U.S. Department of Defense, October 1992.

Maryland.   The U.S. Army Medical Material Development Activity (USAMMDA), with a yearly operating budget of $15 million to $20 million, is DOD's product development unit. USAMMDA supports a clinical testing facility at the University of Maryland, Baltimore, and manufactures pilot lots of vaccines, including those for Q fever, Rift Valley fever, and Venezuelan equine encephalitis, through a contract with the Salk Institute in Swiftwater, Pennsylvania.   DOD completed modernization of its own pilot vaccine manufacturing facility in 1992 at Forest Glen, Maryland, at an estimated cost of $5 million.   This $25 million facility, expected to be fully validated and functional in October 1993, will be capable of producing up to 1 million doses of vaccine for clinical trials annually by using traditional or modern molecular biology techniques (Jerald C. Sadoff, Walter Reed Army Institute of Research, personal communication, 1993).   DOD also supports a number of overseas field laboratories that have the capacity to conduct vaccine-related research on a variety of tropical diseases.   The laboratories are based in Thailand, Kenya, Brazil, Peru, Indonesia, and Egypt.

National Institutes of Health

The National Institutes of Health supports an active program in vaccine research, implemented through intramural research projects and extramural contracts, cooperative research and development agreements, and grants. Although the research is conducted through a number of institutes, including the National Cancer Institute and the National Institute of Child Health and

Human Development (NICHD), the vast majority of vaccine research is concentrated at the National Institute of Allergy and Infectious Diseases (NIAID).

In 1981, NIAID founded its Program for Accelerated Development of Vaccines to focus and enhance research activities leading to new vaccines for important diseases. Over the next decade, the program grew, addressing vaccine priorities with the assistance of previous Institute of Medicine studies (Institute of Medicine, 1986a,b). The 1991 NIH Strategic Plan identified vaccines and immunology as a trans-NIH critical area of technology and provided a framework for strengthening nontraditional targets. The goals of the CVI provide an additional focus for vaccine research and development that combines the goal of prevention with goals that incorporate the availability of vaccines that are more effective and efficient in preventing infectious diseases, both in the United States and abroad.

In 1992, NIAID created the Task Force on Microbiology and Infectious Disease, which provided NIAID with guidance for future research directions in six areas, including the accelerated development of vaccines (National Institute of Allergy and Infectious Diseases, 1992a). Recommendations of the task force included the following: applied vaccine research, including studies on the most effective bacterial or viral carriers, increased temperature stability, improved efficacy and safety of adjuvants, and the development of preparations allowing for the controlled release of immunogens for single-dose vaccines; development of more effective, safer, and preferably, oral vaccines; and production of experimental vaccines on a pilot plant scale and under acceptable conditions for subsequent use in clinical trials (National Institute of Allergy and Infectious Diseases, 1992a).

In addition to traditional grants and contracts, there are several key elements of NIAID's vaccine research program. Extensive portfolios of investigator-initiated research projects in infectious diseases, microbiology, and immunology are complemented by intramural laboratories, collaborations with industry, and research groups that focus, at least in part, on key areas of vaccinology. NIAID supports seven Vaccine and Treatment Evaluation Units (VTEUs), one Mucosal Immunization Group, one Maternal Immunization Group, seven International Collaborations in Infectious Disease Research, three Tropical Medicine Research Centers, five Centers for Sexually Transmitted Diseases, and four Tropical Disease Research Units. Established in the early 1960s to evaluate the safety and immunogenicity of candidate vaccines in human trials, the network of VTEUs is based at university-affiliated medical research facilities in the United States. In addition, NIAID supports (to a more limited extent) the preclinical evaluation of vaccines in animal models and primates as well as the development of reagents and reference serologic assays. NIAID has a

TABLE 3-4 NIAID Vaccine-Related Research

Research Area	Amount Spent (in thousands of $) in Fiscal Year:[a]		
	1991	1992	1993 (estimated)
AIDS	36,026 (33.94)	43,084 (34.13)	45,140 (34.38)
Tropical diseases	6,452 (6.08)	6,745 (5.34)	6,987 (5.32)
R&D on children's diseases	39,003 (36.74)	49,674 (39.35)	51,462 (39.20)
Other	24,670 (23.24)	26,730 (21.12)	27,693 (21.09)
Total	106,151 (100.00)	126,233 (100.00)	131,282 (100.00)

[a] Values in parentheses are the percentage of the total.

SOURCE: S. Berkowitz, National Institute of Allergy and Infectious Diseases, 1992.

limited capacity for production of pilot lots of vaccine under contract. Finally, the clinical evaluation of vaccines is supplemented by a regulatory support infrastructure which the NIAID has developed over the past decades.

In fiscal year 1993, NIAID will spend an estimated $131 million on research related to vaccines—more than any other federal entity (Table 3-4). Of that amount, roughly one-third ($45 million) will go toward work on a vaccine against HIV. Vaccines immunizing against a total of 33 other specific viral, bacterial, or parasitic agents will be targeted in the research, including six (filariae, leishmania, leprosy, malaria, schistosomes, and trypanosomes) investigated as part of the United Nations Development Program/World Bank/WHO Special Program for Research and Training in Tropical Diseases. In fiscal year 1993, an additional $5.3 million was earmarked for research on CVI-related vaccines.

NIAID has no in-house capacity to produce pilot lots of vaccine, but it does have a limited capacity to contract out pilot vaccine production. However, the NICHD does have a very small pilot vaccine production facility at the NIH campus in Bethesda, Maryland. NICHD currently spends approximately $8 million to $9 million on pediatric vaccine-related activities.

National Vaccine Program

Organized efforts to develop a vaccine policy for the United States began during World War II, when the Armed Forces Epidemiology Board planned the vaccine strategies for the war effort. The Office of the Assistant Secretary for Health made efforts to develop a national immunization policy that would ensure progress in vaccine-based disease prevention as early as 1976, following the anticipated swine flu epidemic (Institute of Medicine, 1985). Between 1979 and 1985, the congressional Office of Technology Assessment and the Institute of Medicine both worked to formulate approaches for creating a national vaccine policy (Institute of Medicine, 1985; Office of Technology Assessment, 1979). These efforts were motivated by a recognition that, despite the resources available for vaccine development and immunization, without a strategic plan and management structure, U.S. immunization efforts would continue to fall short of their potential.

The National Vaccine Program (NVP) was created in 1986 by the same law (P.L. 99-660) that authorized the Vaccine Injury Compensation Program (see Appendix F for authorizing legislation). NVP's goal was to achieve optimal protection from infectious diseases in the United States through the use of immunization. The NVP was assigned two functions: to develop a National Vaccine Plan annually and to provide special funds (intended to reach $30 million per year) to federal agencies to complete critical portions of the plan. In addition, an independent National Vaccine Advisory Committee was to be appointed in consultation with the Institute of Medicine. The National Vaccine Plan was supposed to outline the activities needed to advance vaccines from the research and development stage through to field trials, licensing, production, use, and finally, surveillance of adverse effects.

The congressional committee that drafted the legislation believed that a National Vaccine Plan would provide the strongest argument for an infusion of new funds into vaccine and immunization programs. However, the Reagan Administration opposed the National Vaccine Program. No full-time administrator was appointed, and no appropriation was requested for the NVP during its first 3 years (Budget of the U.S. Government, 1987, 1988, 1989; Freeman, 1991; Medicine and Health, 1990). The administration believed that the Department of Health and Human Services could conduct of all the planning envisioned by the legislation with no new statutory authority. No National Vaccine Plan, required annually since January 1, 1987, has been submitted to the U.S. Congress. In the absence of a National Vaccine Plan, appropriations committees in the U.S. Congress have been reluctant to appropriate the funds whose use was to be guided by the plan. The measles epidemic of 1989–1990 underscored the need, however, to plan vaccine and immunization activities in the United States (National Vaccine Advisory Committee, 1991).

By fiscal year 1991, the NVP had a staffing level of 23 FTEs and an operating budget of $9.5 million, most of which was distributed to other federal agencies (U.S. Department of Health and Human Services, 1992). In fiscal year 1991, the largest share of NVPO funds went to the CDC ($3.3

million), including nearly $1.3 million for research activities (U.S. Department of Health and Human Services, 1992). NIH received $2.7 million, almost all of which supported an ongoing trial of an acellular pertussis vaccine. The allocation to FDA totaled $1.9 million, $1 million of which supported research activities. The NVP itself received $1.4 million in fiscal year 1991 for operational expenses, primarily salaries and overhead (U.S. Department of Health and Human Services, 1992). In fiscal year 1992, NVPO funding fell to $7.9 million, and in fiscal year 1993, the appropriation dropped to $2.8 million.

The committee is disturbed by the lack of support for the NVP because it believes that the concept of planning, organizing, and managing existing immunization resources under an accountable government mandate is vital to the development and use of vaccines. There is no doubt that the NVP's planning function and coordination of public-sector activities must be continued into the future. The NVP does not, however, as currently authorized, possess the programmatic nor operational capability to manage the development of new vaccines.

Other Federal Programs

Not all federal investments in immunization go toward purchasing vaccines or research. There are a number of ongoing efforts that have a positive but indirect impact on immunization services. These include initiatives designed to ensure access to immunization services, educate the public about the value of vaccination, and promote the appropriate use of childhood vaccines.

For example, one important goal of Medicaid, the state-administered health program overseen by the Health Care Financing Administration, is to provide regular immunizations for those under age 21. Two programs (the Community and Migrant Health Centers and Maternal and Child Health Block Grant) run by the Health Resources and Services Administration have as a central mandate the provision of immunizations to particularly needy populations. Funds in the Maternal and Child Health Block Grant program are used by the states' local health departments to improve vaccine delivery services. All children participating in Head Start, a program of the Administration for Children and Families, are entitled to receive a comprehensive set of health services, including immunizations (National Vaccine Advisory Committee, 1992).

In cooperation with the CDC, the U.S. Department of Agriculture has mounted an effort to increase immunization coverage among children who receive food under the Supplemental Food Program for Women, Infants, and Children. The U.S. Department of Education is working with federal health officials to improve the availability and accessibility of comprehensive health care, including immunization, for migrant farm workers (National Vaccine Advisory Committee, 1992).

U.S. State Vaccine Manufacturers

Only two public-sector facilities in the United States manufacture selected vaccines for a small subset of the U.S. population. The states of Massachusetts and Michigan manufacture a range of vaccines for their respective residents.

Massachusetts

The Massachusetts Department of Public Health operates a comprehensive state-run vaccine research and production program. Massachusetts' Biologic Laboratories conduct basic and applied research and manufacture bacterial vaccines for the state's immunization program. Massachusetts holds licenses from FDA to manufacture several vaccines, including the combination diphtheria and tetanus toxoid and pertussis vaccine (DTP), combination diphtheria-tetanus toxoids, and combination adult tetanus and diphtheria toxoids. Acellular pertussis and *Haemophilus influenzae* type b vaccines (Hib) are in the clinical development stages. The annual production volume is rarely more than 500,000 doses of each vaccine. Virtually all vaccines are distributed within Massachusetts, although the laboratories have several agreements with commercial companies for collaborative vaccine development.

The laboratories' annual operating budget is about $8 million, which consists of $1 million in state appropriated funds and revenues from the sale and licensing of biologics such as varcilla-zoster immune globulin and cytomegalovirus immune globulin. By statute, Massachusetts can be sued for torts, but liability is limited to $100,000 per claim (George Siber, Massachusetts Biologics Laboratories, personal communication, 1993).

Michigan

Like Massachusetts, the laboratories of the Michigan Department of Public Health develop and manufacture vaccines primarily for in-state use. On average, 700,000 doses of DTP are produced annually, although the capacity for DTP production is many times that (Robert Myers, Michigan

Biologics Laboratories, personal communication, 1993). The state's annual appropriation for the Biologics Laboratories is roughly $3 million per year, approximately one-fourth to one-third the facility's total operating budget. Other revenues are derived through Cooperative Research and Development Agreements, the licensing of several products, and the sale on a cost-recovery basis of several vaccines; among them are sales to the DOD.

In addition to DTP, Michigan is licensed to produce tetanus toxoid, adsorbed; diphtheria and tetanus toxoids, adsorbed; pertussis vaccine, adsorbed; rabies vaccine, adsorbed; and anthrax vaccine, adsorbed. Each component is manufactured in a separate facility, enabling simultaneous production. Products that Michigan is currently working on include an acellular pertussis component, a combination DTP-hepatitis B vaccine, and a combination DTP-hepatitis B-Hib vaccine; two of these products are being developed through collaborative efforts with SmithKline Beecham. Because of a judicial "clarification of sovereign immunity," state-produced vaccines are largely immune from tort action in Michigan (Robert Myers, Michigan Biologics Laboratories, personal communication, 1993).

U.S.-Based Pharmaceutical Firms

Only a handful of private-sector companies in the United States currently manufacture pediatric vaccines for the U.S. population.

Connaught Laboratories, Inc.

Connaught Laboratories, Inc., in Swiftwater, Pennsylvania, is a wholly owned subsidiary of Connaught Laboratories Ltd., of Toronto, Canada. Connaught Laboratories Limited has, since 1989, been a subsidiary of Pasteur Mérieux Sérums et Vaccins, which is 51 percent owned by Rhône-Poulenc, a highly diversified French chemical and pharmaceutical company which is partially held by the government of France.

Connaught manufactures and distributes vaccines against polio (made with inactivated poliovirus), diphtheria, tetanus, pertussis, and *Haemophilus influenzae* type b. The company has a number of other vaccines in various stages of development, including a Lyme disease vaccine, a meningococcal group B vaccine (for those 2 years of age and older), a pneumococcal conjugate vaccine, a hepatitis B vaccine, and an acellular pertussis DTP-Hib conjugate combination-hepatitis B vaccine. This company was also recently licensed to produce a Japanese encephalitis vaccine. Several other Product License Applications have been submitted to the FDA by Connaught

Laboratories (Douglas Reynolds, Connaught Laboratories, Inc., personal communication, 1992).

Lederle-Praxis Biologicals

Employing approximately 600 people, Lederle-Praxis Biologicals is a division of the American Cyanamid Company—a major chemical company in the United States that derived over half of its 1990 total sales from its Medical Group, which includes pharmaceuticals, biologics, and medical devices and supplies (Hoover et al., 1991). In 1989, American Cyanamid's Lederle Laboratories acquired Praxis Biologics, a biotechnology firm that had developed a *Haemophilus influenzae* type b vaccine (Hib).

Lederle-Praxis is the first company in the United States to market an acellular pertussis vaccine for use as a booster in older infants and young children. In March 1993, the FDA licensed Lederle-Praxis' combination DTP-Hib for use in infants. This marked the first combination vaccine to be licensed in the United States since MMR was licensed in 1971. Other Lederle-Praxis Biologicals' licensed products include two Hib conjugate vaccines (licensed for administration at different ages), oral polio vaccine, and DTP. Products in the development pipeline include a respiratory syncytial virus vaccine and a Sabin inactivated polio vaccine (Jane Scott, Lederle-Praxis Biologicals, personal communication, 1992; Pharmaceutical Manufacturers Association, 1990). Lederle-Praxis Biologicals, which has traditionally focused exclusively on the U.S. market, has recently sought to license its products in Europe and the Confederation of Independent States (Frank Cano, Lederle-Praxis Biologicals, personal communication, 1992).

Merck & Co., Inc.

Merck & Co., Inc., is a 100-year-old chemical and pharmaceutical company headquartered in Rahway, New Jersey. Merck currently manufactures six vaccines: hepatitis B, Hib, measles, mumps, rubella, and several combination products made from these components. The most widely used is the measles, mumps, and rubella (MMR) combination. The firm has a number of vaccines in the development pipeline (see Chapter 4). Two vaccines are close to FDA approval: a varicella (chicken pox) vaccine is undergoing FDA review for licensure, and a hepatitis A vaccine is in phase III clinical trials (Glenna Crooks, Merck & Co, Inc., personnal communication, 1993; Merck & Co., Inc., 1991a; Pharmaceutical Manufacturers Association, 1990).

In 1989, Merck signed an agreement with the People's Republic of China under which the company will provide the technology needed to produce its recombinant hepatitis B vaccine. Merck trained teams of Chinese engineers, production personnel, and quality control specialists, who will then train additional staff at production plants in Beijing and Shenzhen. The training program ended in mid-1992, at which time the production equipment was shipped to China (Glenna Crooks, Merck & Co, Inc., personnal communication, 1993; Merck & Co., Inc., 1991a).

In April 1991, Merck created a separate vaccine division, noting its "commitment to vaccines, which are so important to world healthcare but have been abandoned by some pharmaceutical firms" (Merck & Co., Inc., 1991a). Two months later, the company signed a collaborative agreement with Connaught Laboratories, Inc., an affiliate of Pasteur Mérieux Sérums et Vaccins, to develop and market pediatric vaccines containing multiple antigens, including DTP, Hib, hepatitis B, and inactivated poliomyelitis in the United States. In 1993, Merck & Co., Inc., and Pasteur Mérieux Sérums et Vaccins signed an agreement forming a joint venture to market vaccine products in Europe and to develop pediatric combination vaccines containing these same multiple antigens. Sales of vaccine (human and animal) and other biologics accounted for approximately 5 percent of Merck's total sales in 1990 (Merck & Co., Inc., 1991b).

SmithKline Beecham

SmithKline Beecham (SB) is among the world's largest pharmaceutical companies, with 1991 sales of $8.8 billion (SmithKline Beecham, 1991). SB markets its products to 130 countries and is actively involved in the development of multicomponent vaccines. SB's primary activities include the development, manufacture, and marketing of both human and animal pharmaceuticals and biologics, as well as clinical laboratory testing services. SB's hepatitis B vaccine enjoyed a rapid increase in sales (25 percent) in 1991 over the previous year (SmithKline Beecham, 1991). In addition, the world's first hepatitis A vaccine was approved in the vaccine's first markets–Switzerland and Belgium–in 1991. As of the beginning of 1992, SB had both an improved pertussis vaccine and an improved polio vaccine in phase III clinical trials. Although the company produces a number of vaccines, only its hepatitis B vaccine is approved for sale in the United States. As noted above, SB is currently collaborating with the Michigan Department of Public Health on several vaccine products, including combination vaccines. SB's vaccine manufacturing facility is based in Rixensart, Belgium; there are no human vaccine manufacturing facilities in the United States at this time.

Wyeth-Ayerst

Wyeth-Ayerst is a division of American Home Products Corporation, a 48,000-employee company headquartered in Madison, New Jersey. Wyeth-Ayerst manufactures influenza, cholera, typhoid, and adenovirus vaccines, and diphtheria toxoid. In 1991, phase III clinical trials of a rotavirus vaccine were being conducted as part of a Cooperative Research and Development Agreement with the National Institutes of Health. Also in 1991, Investigational New Drug (IND) applications were filed with the FDA for a cold-adapted, nasally delivered influenza vaccine (licensed from the University of Michigan) and another influenza vaccine (utilizing an adjuvant system licensed from Syntex) intended for use in the elderly. IND submissions were planned for several new oral hepatitis B vaccines, and laboratory research and preclinical testing were being conducted on a potential vaccine for Lyme disease (American Home Products, 1991).

Development-Stage Companies

A number of small start-up and biotechnology firms based in the United States are actively involved in vaccine research and development. With a few exceptions, these companies have no vaccine products on the market. Most firms have directed their efforts to developing vaccines of need in the United States and the industrialized world. The firms discussed below are meant to illustrate the kinds of activities undertaken by these smaller companies. Nothing about the relative merits of these companies in comparison with those of companies not discussed here should be inferred from this list, nor should this list be seen as an endorsement of any one firm's operations.

North American Vaccine

North American Vaccine (NAV) is a biotechnology company with research and production facilities in Beltsville, Maryland. In 1991, phase III clinical testing of the company's acellular pertussis vaccine (in combination with diphtheria vaccine and tetanus toxoids) was in progress. The trial was being conducted in Sweden under the sponsorship of the National Institute of Child Health and Human Development. NAV is conducting preclinical and clinical research on a number of potential vaccine products, including a DTP-inactivated polio vaccine and vaccines intended to prevent meningitis, group B streptococcus, and otitis media. In 1991, NAV had $889,000 in contract revenue and posted a $5.8 million operating loss for the year. The company raised nearly $44 million in 1991 through a public stock offering (North American Vaccine, 1991).

MedImmune

Based in Gaithersburg, Maryland, MedImmune has a worldwide exclusive license for the use of recombinant BCG (bacillus Calmette-Guérin) as a carrier for vaccination against human and animal diseases. The company has two recombinant BCG vaccines (against AIDS and Lyme disease) in preclinical studies. MedImmune is collaborating with Merck on the AIDS vaccine and with Connaught Laboratories, Inc., on the Lyme disease vaccine. A number of other BCG-based vaccines–against pneumococcal pneumonia, hepatitis B, malaria, and schistosomiasis–are undergoing preclinical testing. MedImmune also is working to develop a multivalent childhood vaccine that uses the same technology of BCG as a vector.

In 1991, MedImmune had $5.6 million in sales from the one product it had on the market, an immune serum called CytoGam. The firm brought in another $8.3 million through outside research and licensing agreements and invested $7.7 million in research and development (MedImmune, Inc., 1991).

Univax Biologics, Inc.

Univax Biologics, Inc., a small biotechnology firm located in Rockville, Maryland, has as its primary research and development focus the development of hyperimmune intravenous immunoglobulins. Three vaccines used to stimulate antibody production for intravenous immunoglobulin therapy were in phase II trials in 1991, and two others were expected to enter phase I studies in 1992.

The company has plans to develop two of its antisepsis vaccines: for use as vaccines one, against *Staphylococcus aureus*, for use in kidney dialysis patients; the other, a synthetic conjugate vaccine against endotoxin, intended to prevent septic shock. Univax is also developing a recombinant DNA-produced vaccine against HIV (UNIVAX Biologics, Inc., 1992).

Univax' 1991 revenues totaled nearly $1.3 million, almost all of which was income from research and development agreements. The company spent $4.5 million on its own research in 1991, and had a net operating loss of $4.3 million. In February 1992, Univax raised $44 million through a public stock offering (UNIVAX Biologics, Inc., 1992).

Nongovernmental Organizations

The Children's Defense Fund

The Children's Defense Fund (CDF) is a Washington, D.C.-based nonprofit lobbying and educational organization. Founded in 1973 by Marian Wright Edelman, CDF has as its mandate the improvement of living conditions for the nation's children. A significant amount of the group's efforts is directed toward health issues, including the promotion of immunization in the United States. CDF publishes a number of reports each year. These are intended to inform and influence public opinion related to child health issues (Children's Defense Fund, undated).

March of Dimes Birth Defects Foundation

Founded by President Franklin D. Roosevelt in 1938 as the National Foundation for Infantile Paralysis to fight polio in the United States, the organization was later renamed the March of Dimes Birth Defects Foundation (MOD). Its mission is to improve the health of infants through prevention of birth defects and infant mortality, recognizing the key role of vaccines in improving infant health. MOD vigorously supports basic and applied research and granted over $20 million to over 600 grantees in 1991. Other areas of activity include community outreach services (clinics, hotlines, and special programs), health education for parents expecting a child, and advocacy for state and national legislation concerning maternal, prenatal, and child health (March of Dimes Birth Defects Foundation, 1991).

Rockefeller Foundation

Located in New York City, the Rockefeller Foundation is one of the oldest and largest philanthropic entities in the United States. Although it provides grants in many different areas, the foundation has targeted three primary areas, one of which is international science-based development. Included in this sphere is its commitment to disease prevention through vaccinology and pharmacology. In 1990, the Rockefeller Foundation's health sciences program expenditures totaled $14 million, representing 15 percent of total expenditures. In 1991, the foundation appropriated nearly $1 million to vaccine production technology transfer activities, attempting to make viral vaccine production a more generic and technically accessible process that would be available at affordable cost to developing countries. In addition, the Rockefeller Foundation awards numerous grants for vaccine development projects all over the world, with a special emphasis on diseases in the developing world. The Rockefeller Foundation has been a major contributor to the EPI research and development program, the WHO/United Nations Development Program/Program for Vaccine Development, and is one of the four founders of the global CVI. The Rockefeller Foundation was once a research organization in its own right and is credited with the development of the yellow fever vaccine and the transfer of its manufacture to Brazil (Rockefeller Foundation, 1991).

Rotary Foundation

The Rotary Foundation, established by Rotary International in 1917, is an educational and charitable endowment. Since 1985, the foundation has raised over $240 million to support worldwide efforts to eradicate polio. The Rotary initiative PolioPlus has made grants to nearly 100 developing countries for the purchase of polio vaccine from the United Nations Children's Fund and Pan American Health Organization sources. Rotary International was among the first donors to support the CVI by providing funds for the product development group on a heat-stable oral polio vaccine (OPV). The Rotary Foundation is also supporting the People's Republic of China's OPV plant. Rotarians and Rotary Clubs around the world participate to varying degrees in polio immunization and surveillance activities (Rotary Foundation of Rotary International, undated).

* * *

The U.S. public sector devotes over $250 million to various aspects of vaccine research and development (Table 3-5). Comparable figures for U.S. private sector-investments (commercial vaccine manufacturers and newly emerging biotechnology firms) in vaccine research and development are unavailable. However, commercial vaccine manufacturers likely invest between 12 and 15 percent of their total vaccine sales in vaccine research and development. The U.S. vaccine market, which is dominated by a handful of firms, has been estimated to range between $500 million and $800 million (Cohen, 1993). As such, it is likely that commercial vaccine manufacturers in the United States invest approximately $100 million in vaccine research and development on an annual basis. The investment of biotechnology firms in vaccine research and development is unknown.

TABLE 3-5 Pubic-Sector Expenditures for Vaccine Research and Development in the United States

Entity	1992 Expenditure (in millions of $)	Funds or Conducts R&D
AID	15.0[a]	Funds
CBER/FDA	14.9	Conducts
DOD	76.7	Conducts
Massachusetts	1.5	Conducts
Michigan	1.5	Conducts
NCID/CDC	2.1[b]	Conducts
NIAID/NIH	126.2	Funds/Conducts
NICHD/NIH	8.0	Funds/Conducts
NVP	7.9	Funds
Total	253.8	

[a] This figure represents 1991 funding.
[b] This figure represents pediatric vaccines only.

Despite the substantial number of U.S. government agencies, private firms, and other organizations involved in vaccine-related activities, and despite specific legislation mandating a National Vaccine Plan, there has been no overall strategy guiding the research, production, procurement, and distribution of childhood vaccines in the United States. As noted in a recent Institute of Medicine report, ". . . the overall process of vaccine development, manufacturing, and use in the United States is fragmented. There is no direct connection between research and development on the one hand and use of vaccines on the other. The various decision makers do not work together; in fact, they respond to different pressures" (Institute of Medicine, 1992, p. 157). As a result, the system of vaccine development and supply lacks a certain degree of cohesion. For example, in the current system, costly research and development performed in the private sector are not always done in conjunction with what the public sector might identify as the greatest public health needs. Similarly and with specific regard to the CVI, U.S. government agencies interact with the global CVI virtually independently of each other.

INTERNATIONAL RESOURCES

Numerous multilateral and bilateral organizations support aspects of vaccine research, development, manufacture, procurement, or distribution. The following sections focus primarily on multilateral organizations.

Multilateral Organizations

Pan American Health Organization

The Pan American Health Organization (PAHO) is a public health agency that serves as a regional office of WHO. PAHO raises money to assist its 38 member countries in carrying out health programs, disseminates scientific and technical information throughout the inter-American region, trains health-care workers and strengthens national training institutions, and hires scientific and technical experts to address priority health issues in Latin America and the Caribbean (Pan American Health Organization, undated).

PAHO Revolving Fund During the 1970s, countries in the Americas faced considerable difficulties raising hard currency to purchase needed pediatric vaccines for their Expanded Program on Immunization programs. In response to this problem, in 1979 PAHO established a revolving fund for the purchase of vaccines and related supplies for EPI in the Americas. The revolving fund has a working capital of $5.5 million. Member countries pay local currency equivalents for vaccine purchases, and PAHO pays for the vaccine using hard currency from the fund. Local currency is channeled back into a variety of operations and programs in the country (Ciro de Quadros, Pan American Health Organization, personal communication, 1993).

SIREVA Project The Regional System for Vaccines in the Americas (SIREVA) was established in 1991 as a possible model for collaboration among developing countries for vaccine research and production activities. SIREVA is a multinational system designed to generate epidemiological knowledge related to vaccine development and identify, develop, and evaluate candidate vaccines of importance to the region. SIREVA's first vaccine research and development projects are targeted against three diseases of prevalence in the Americas: pneumococcal disease in children, typhoid fever, and meningitis due to *Haemophilus influenzae* type b organisms. Whenever possible, the data and technologies acquired through SIREVA will remain in the public domain. It is hoped that SIREVA will eventually become an administratively and financially independent operation (Pan American Health Organization, 1991).

United Nations Development Program

The United Nations Development Program (UNDP) is the largest multilateral grant assistance organization in the world. It plays a key coordinating role for development activities undertaken by the United Nations. UNDP focuses its efforts in six priority areas: poverty alleviation and grass roots development, environment and natural resources, management development, technical cooperation, technology transfer, and women in development. Among other initiatives, UNDP actively supports the CVI, EPI, the Global Program on AIDS, the WHO/UNDP Program for Vaccine Development (described below), and the UNDP/World Bank/WHO Special Program for Research and Development in Tropical Diseases. Financed by voluntary contributions from governments, $1.4 billion was pledged to UNDP from member nations in 1991 (United Nations Development Program, 1992). UNDP is currently exploring the possibility of setting up an international vaccine institute in East Asia to facilitate improvements in vaccine quality and to promote technology transfer.

United Nations Children's Fund

UNICEF plays a critical role in enhancing immunization activities throughout the world through its purchases of vaccine, provision of cold-chain equipment and other supplies, training of health-care workers, and provision of resources to assist with social mobilization efforts. UNICEF currently buys about half of the vaccine used in EPI programs and has spent over $500 million on immunization since 1982, including approximately $177 million on vaccine purchases (UNICEF, 1991). In 1992, UNICEF procured $65 million worth of vaccine. In addition to its core activities, UNICEF plays a strong advocacy role promoting immunization programs around the world.

In the next 5 years, over 5.5 billion doses of vaccine costing $363 million will be needed to maintain EPI programs around the world (UNICEF, 1991). About 10 countries have requested UNICEF assistance in procuring hepatitis B vaccine (John Gilmartin, UNICEF, personal communication, 1993). Given this level of need and current resources, there is likely to be a significant shortfall in the amount of vaccine available for EPI activities (UNICEF, 1991; World Health Organization/Children's Vaccine Initiative, 1992b).

Vaccine Independence Initiative The Vaccine Independence Initiative was launched in early 1992 in an effort to help countries become self-sufficient purchasers of vaccine (UNICEF, 1991). Under the initiative, which is modeled after the PAHO revolving fund, UNICEF buys vaccine for the country and the country pays UNICEF the local currency equivalent for the vaccine. UNICEF then uses the local currency to administer UNICEF

programs in the country. Among its other goals, the initiative is designed
to help countries forecast vaccine budgets and coordinate the immunization
activities of various national ministries. Initial capital support for the
Vaccine Independence Initiative has been provided by the U.S. Agency for
International Development. In June 1992, the Kingdom of Morocco became
the first country to participate in the Vaccine Independence Initiative
(World Health Organization/Children's Vaccine Initiative, 1992b).

World Bank

The World Bank, officially known as the International Bank for
Reconstruction and Development, was established in 1945 to help rebuild
countries that were devastated during World War II. ˙ Owned by 160
governments, the principal purpose of the World Bank today is to raise the
standard of living in developing countries by using resources from
industrialized countries. In its early years, the World Bank primarily
supported infrastructure projects such as road building and the construction
of power-generating plants and telecommunications networks (World Bank,
1992).

Since 1973, in an effort to benefit the citizens of developing countries
more directly, World Bank lending is now targeted toward agricultural and
rural development, education, health, nutrition, family planning, housing and
urban services, water resources development, and electrification. The Bank
is founding member of the UNDP/World Bank/WHO Special Program for
Research and Training on Tropical Diseases, as well as a founding but
nonpaying member of the CVI. It is currently financing a project in the
People's Republic of China to build new vaccine manufacturing facilities for
DTP, oral polio vaccine, and measles vaccine.

World Health Organization

Created in 1948, WHO is an intergovernmental organization within the
United Nations system that is responsible for coordinating and directing
international public health matters. The WHO executes its work through
three principal bodies: the World Health Assembly, an annual meeting to
discuss WHO's program plan and attended by delegates from the 166
member states; the Executive Board, comprising 31 individuals designated
by member states; and the Secretariat, which is staffed by some 4,500 health
experts under the leadership of a Director-General and which is responsible
for overseeing the day-to-day operations of WHO. There are six WHO
regional offices worldwide. The 1992–1993 operating budget of the WHO

totaled approximately $1.7 billion, an increase of .3 billion from the 1990-1991 budget (Budget Office, World Health Organization, Washington, D.C., personal communication, 1993).

Expanded Program on Immunization EPI was established by the World Health Assembly in May 1974 to assist national immunization programs in the developing world. To date, the EPI has been enormously successful in increasing immunization coverage among children in the developing world (see Chapter 2).

In order to advance the long-term goal of universal childhood immunization, EPI supports a number of different activities related to vaccine delivery and utilization. These include the production of training and educational materials; assistance in planning and evaluating national immunization programs; surveillance of global, regional, and national immunization coverage and disease data; and promotion of the research and development necessary to solve operational problems. Although they may receive assistance from the EPI, national governments are ultimately responsible for coordinating and implementing their respective immunization programs. The EPI's operating budget for 1992–1993 totaled $30,325,600, falling from its 1990–1991 level of $46,019,700. Approximately $11 million of the 1992–1993 budget was allocated directly overseas, while roughly $19 million was appropriated to global and interregional funds to be disbursed by the Geneva headquarters (Budget Office, World Health Organization, Washington, DC, personal communication, 1993).

Program for Vaccine Development The Program for Vaccine Development (PVD), which was initiated by the Director-General of WHO in 1984, coordinates international vaccine development with academic institutions and other scientific groups and encourages the participation and training of scientists from developing countries. Since its founding, PVD has trained over 500 scientists from 87 countries. PVD activities are guided by the Scientific Advisory Group of Experts, an international group of vaccine specialists. In 1990, PVD became a partnership between WHO and UNDP.

By the end of 1991, PVD had received nearly $22 million in outside contributions from such groups as the Rockefeller Foundation, the Glenmede Trust, UNDP, and the governments of Australia, France, Italy, Japan, Norway, Sweden, and Switzerland. In 1991, the PVD budget was $5.9 million and the organization supported a total of 94 vaccine development projects in 22 countries (World Health Organization, 1991). In 1992, however, the budget fell to $4.9 million (World Health Organization/Children's Vaccine Initiative, 1993).

Children's Vaccine Initiative The CVI, both a concept and an organization, is an international effort to accelerate the application of modern science and technology to the development of new and better childhood vaccines. The ultimate goal of the CVI, which was established following the 1990 World Summit for Children in New York City, is to develop a means of immunizing children at birth against all important childhood diseases. The desirable features of CVI vaccines are that they be given in a single dose, administered near birth, combined in novel ways, heat stable, effective against a variety of diseases, and affordable. The activities of CVI are carried out primarily through product development groups and task forces (see Chapter 2).

The CVI is cosponsored by five organizations: UNICEF, UNDP, the Rockefeller Foundation, the World Bank, and WHO. The CVI is financed from voluntary contributions from governments, foundations, and international organizations. In 1992, the CVI budget stood at $3.8 million. The estimated budget for 1993 is $6.5 million (World Health Organization/Children's Vaccine Initiative, 1992a).

Public-Sector Resources

Many countries maintain public-sector institutes or support facilities that manufacture vaccines. Most often, the primary goal of such efforts is to meet the vaccine needs of the citizens of the respective country. Some countries manufacture all of their childhood vaccines, others import components for the manufacture of vaccines, and yet others purchase and import bulk vaccine for subsequent finishing and processing. The National Institute of Public Health and Environmental Protection (Rijksinstituut voor Volksgezondheid en Milieuhygiene) in The Netherlands manufactures DTP, inactivated polio vaccine, and MMR (see the box on RIVM in The Netherlands). State Bacteriological Laboratories in Sweden and the State Serum Institute of Denmark also import or produce vaccines that are deemed necessary for their respective national immunization programs. In eastern Europe, Czechoslovakia (now the Czech Republic and Slovakia) and Hungary manufacture a limited number of primarily bacterial vaccines. The Oswaldo Cruz Foundation in Brazil produces a number of different vaccines, including tetanus toxoid, DTP, and measles vaccine for the Brazilian population. Taiwan, India, Indonesia, and the People's Republic of China also produce some of the vaccines required by their respective populations.

Not all of the countries that produce vaccines are self-sufficient in all or even one of the vaccines required by that country, however. Indeed, many countries, particularly those in the developing world, do not have the capacity to meet local demand and so must import vaccine either directly from the manufacturer or through such mechanisms as the PAHO revolving fund or UNICEF. For example, although Egypt's vaccine production institute, Vaccsera, makes tetanus toxoid, DTP, and BCG and imports bulk oral polio vaccine and hepatitis B vaccine for further finishing and packaging, Egypt is unable to produce enough of any single vaccine to meet national demand and obtains the remainder through UNICEF.

Unlike private-sector companies, most public-sector operations have neither the budget nor the capacity to conduct extensive research and development and must acquire vaccine-related technology elsewhere. One of the critical problems for many national institutes in both industrialized and developing countries is obtaining the seed stock and the necessary production technology to manufacture a given vaccine (Homma, 1992). For those countries that possess basic vaccine production equipment, upgrading and improving that technology has proven to be an equally great problem. In 1980, for example, Brazil received second-generation measles vaccine production technology from Japan. The measles vaccine has improved significantly and is now in its fourth generation, yet Brazil has been unable to gain access to this improved vaccine production technology (Homma and Knouss, 1992).

Private-Sector Resources

As of 1992, seven private European vaccine manufacturers produced the majority of vaccines used by Europe and much of the rest of the world. These are Behringwerke (Germany), Immuno (Austria), Medeva-Evans (United Kingdom), Pasteur Mérieux Sérums et Vaccins (France), Sclavo (Italy), SmithKline Beecham (United Kingdom), and Swiss Serum and Vaccine Institute (Switzerland). In 1991, these seven companies formed the European Vaccine Manufacturers, a special group within the European Federation of Pharmaceutical Industries Association. In March 1992, they organized the First European Conference on Vaccinology, in Annecy, France (Baudrihaye, 1992).

Pasteur Mérieux Sérums et Vaccins and SmithKline Beecham are the two largest international suppliers of vaccine, as well as the largest suppliers of vaccine to UNICEF. Pasteur Mérieux Sérums et Vaccins is wholly dedicated to the development of vaccines and biologics. On a much smaller scale is the Swiss Serum and Vaccine Institute, a privately held company that manufactures vaccines for Switzerland and UNICEF.

There has been considerable movement in the pharmaceutical industry in Europe and Asia over the past several years, characterized by a number

National Institute of Public Health and Environmental Protection (RIVM), The Netherlands

RIVM is a Directorate-General of The Netherlands Ministry of Public Health. The primary objective of RIVM's vaccine department is to develop and produce vaccines for the population of The Netherlands; therefore, research, development, and manufacture are generally confined to diseases relevant to The Netherlands' public health and production needs. Development of new vaccines for the developing world and technology transfer have until now been identified as priority tasks of the RIVM, although so far all activities in this respect must be externally funded.

RIVM has pilot facilities for both bacterial and viral vaccines. In 1991, production levels were as follows: DTP, 3 million doses; inactivated polio vaccine, 5 million doses; and MMR, 400,000 doses. Although RIVM does have the capability and capacity to regularly manufacture approximately 18 different vaccines, present policy is to gradually halt production of vaccines that are not relevant to the Netherlands Immunization Program.

Technology transfer activities and capacities are devoted largely to the China Vaccine Project (funded by the World Bank and Rotary International), which is attempting to establish a large scale production capacity for DTP, tetanus toxoids, oral polio vaccine, and measles vaccine in the People's Republic of China through joint development, training, and technology transfer. Another ongoing project involves the upgrading and modernization of DTP production and quality control in Indonesia (this activity is supported by a loan from the Dutch government). In addition, at the request of WHO, RIVM organizes regular quality control courses (mostly focused on polio vaccine) in various countries. Finally, on October 25, 1990, a letter of intent was signed between the National Public Health Institutes of The Netherlands (RIVM), Sweden, Denmark, Norway, and Finland to jointly develop vaccines and transfer vaccine technology to developing countries. The development of a pneumococcal vaccine was selected as a first priority under this Dutch-Nordic Consortium.

Source: A. R. Bergen, Head, Bureau for International Cooperation, RIVM, personal communication, 1992.

of mergers, acquisitions, and joint ventures. Ciba-Geigy, an established pharmaceutical firm based in Switzerland, joined with the U.S. biotechnology company Chiron to form Biocine, which subsequently acquired Sclavo, a medium-sized Italian vaccine manufacturer and supplier of vaccines to UNICEF. Pasteur Mérieux Sérums et Vaccins acquired Connaught Laboratories Ltd., of Canada in 1990. Medeva plc, based in the United Kingdom, bought the vaccine business of Wellcome plc of the United Kingdom in 1991. Medeva is currently the principal vaccine supplier to the National Health Service in the United Kingdom.

Nongovernmental Organizations

Finally, several international nongovernmental organizations support key aspects of immunization programs around the world.

Task Force for Child Survival and Development

Formed in 1984, the Task Force for Child Survival and Development is supported by the World Health Organization, UNICEF, the World Bank, the United Nations Development Program, and the Rockefeller Foundation. The initial mission was to assist in accelerating global childhood immunization. The goals that came out of the 1990 World Summit for Children led to the extension of the task force's mission to address problems concerning nutrition, respiratory infections, diarrheal diseases, breast-feeding, and the Safe Motherhood Initiative, in addition to immunization. Current projects being carried out by the task force include vaccine evaluation efforts in Mexico and Senegal, a surveillance improvement project in Uganda, collaborative neonatal tetanus immunization activities in Bangladesh and Pakistan, and consultation with several countries to help implement effective child survival programs. Barriers to vaccination for children and mothers in developing countries are among the areas of applied research on which the task force is focusing (Task Force for Child Survival and Development, undated).

Save the Children Fund

Founded in 1919, the Save the Children Fund reaches over 50 developing countries as well as the United Kingdom. It has been a strong supporter of the EPI since its inception and has provided vaccines, cold-chain equipment, training materials, technical advisers, and operations research support, as well as conferences and sponsorships. The Save the Children Fund has recently extended its goal to the establishment of sustainable delivery systems for a broad range of basic health services, which includes vaccines (Poore, 1992). Medicins sans Frontieres (Doctors without Borders, France) and the Task Force on Hepatitis B Immunization (based in the United States) are other examples of nongovernmental organizations that continue to influence immunization programs worldwide.

REFERENCES

American Home Products. 1991. Annual Report. Madison, New Jersey.

Baudrihaye N. 1992. European vaccine manufacturers: Present status and future trends. Vaccine 10:893–895.

Budget of the U.S. Government. 1987. Washington, D.C.: U.S. Government Printing Office.

Budget of the U.S. Government. 1988. Washington, D.C: U.S. Government Printing Office.

Budget of the U.S. Government. 1989. Washington, D.C: U.S. Government Printing Office.

Center for Biologics Evaluation and Research, Office of Management. 1993. Data regarding CBER FTEs and budget. Provided in response to Institute of Medicine request. Rockville, Maryland.

Centers for Disease Control and Prevention, Division of Immunization. 1992. Data regarding CDC budget. Provided in response to Institute of Medicine request. Atlanta.

Children's Defense Fund. Undated. General information. Washington, D.C.

Cohen J. 1993. Childhood vaccines: The R&D factor. Science 259:1528–1529.

Freeman P. 1991. Memo to Friends of the National Vaccine Program. The Vaccine Project. March 15. Law Center, University of Massachusetts at Boston.

Homma A. 1992. Technology transfer. Paper presented to the CVI Task Force on Priority Setting and Strategic Plans. Geneva: Children's Vaccine Initiative, Geneva.

Homma A Knouss RF. 1992. Transfer of vaccine technology to developing countries: The Latin American experience. Paper presented at the NIAID Conference on Vaccines and Public Health: Assessing Technologies and Global Policies for the Children's Vaccine Initiative. November 5–6, 1992, Bethesda, Maryland.

Hoover G, Campbell A, Spain PJ, eds. 1991. Hoover's Handbook of American Business 1992. Emeryville, California: The Reference Press.

Institute of Medicine. 1985. Vaccine Supply and Innovation. Washington, D.C.: National Academy Press.

Institute of Medicine. 1986a. New Vaccine Development, Establishing Priorities. Volume I. Diseases of Importance in the United States. Washington, D.C.: National Academy Press.

Institute of Medicine. 1986b. New Vaccine Development, Establishing Priorities. Volume II. Diseases of Importance in the Developing World. Washington, D.C.: National Academy Press.

Institute of Medicine. 1991. Malaria: Obstacles and Opportunities. Washington, D.C.: National Academy Press.

Institute of Medicine. 1992. Emerging Infections. Washington, D.C.: National Academy Press.

Kessler DA. 1992. Testimony before Senate Subcommittee on Labor, Health and Human Services, Committee on Appropriations. Childhood Vaccine Research and Development Issues. April. Washington, D.C: U.S. Congress, Senate.

March of Dimes Birth Defects Foundation. 1991. Annual Report. Washington, D.C.

Medicine and Health. 1990. A shot in the arm for vaccine advocates. Perspectives. July 30. Washington, D.C.

MedImmune, Inc. 1991. Annual Report. Gaithersburg, Maryland.

Merck & Co., Inc. 1991a. Annual Report. Rahway, New Jersey.

Merck & Co., Inc. 1991b. Form 10-K. Washington, D.C.: Securities and Exchange Commission.

National Institute of Allergy and Infectious Diseases. 1992a. Report of the Task Force on Microbiology and Infectious Disease. April. Bethesda, Maryland.

National Institute of Allergy and Infectious Diseases. 1992b. The Jordan Report. Bethesda, Maryland.

National Vaccine Advisory Committee. 1992. Access to Childhood Immunizations: Recommendations and Strategies for Action. April. Rockville, Maryland.

North American Vaccine. 1991. Annual Report. Beltsville, Maryland.

Office of Technology Assessment. 1979. A Review of Selected Federal Vaccine and Immunization Policies. September. Washington, D.C.

Pan American Health Organization. Undated. General information. Washington, D.C.

Pan American Health Organization. 1991. Regional System for Vaccines (SIREVA) Feasibility Study. Washington, D.C.

Pharmaceutical Manufacturers Association. 1990. New Medicines in Development for Children. Fall. Washington, D.C.

Poore P. 1992. Availability of quality vaccines: Policies of a non-governmental organization. Vaccine 10:958–960.

Rockefeller Foundation. 1991. Annual Report. New York, New York.

Rotary Foundation of Rotary International. Undated. PolioPlus. Evanston, Illinois.

SmithKline Beecham. 1991. Annual Report. Philadelphia.

Task Force for Child Survival and Development. Undated. General information. Atlanta.

UNICEF. 1991. Executive Board Action Item: Establishment of a Vaccine Independence Initiative. March 12. New York, New York.

UNICEF. 1992. Vaccine Independence Initiative. Project Proposal for Funding by Interested Donors. July 13. New York, New York.

United Nations Development Program. 1992. New York, New York.

UNIVAX Biologics, Inc. 1992. Common Stock Prospectus. February 4. Rockville, Maryland.

U.S. Agency for International Development. 1992. Overview of Activities Supportive of the Children's Vaccine Initiative. Washington, D.C.

U.S. Department of Defense. Army. Office of the Surgeon General. Health Measures and Immunizations, Preventive Medicine in World War II. Washington, D.C.

U.S. Department of Health and Human Services. 1992. Report on NVPO Expenditures for Acellular Pertussis Vaccine Research and Other Activities. January. Washington, D.C.

World Bank. 1992. Annual Report. Washington, D.C.

World Health Organization. 1991. Programme for Vaccine Development: a WHO/UNDP Partnership. December. Geneva.

World Health Organization. 1992. EPI for the 1990s. Geneva.

World Health Organization/Children's Vaccine Initiative. 1993. Global Investment in Children's Vaccine Research and Development: Results of a Survey. April. Geneva.

World Health Organization/Children's Vaccine Initiative. 1992a. Core Budget and Programme of Work for 1992 and 1993. October. Geneva.

World Health Organization/Children's Vaccine Initiative. 1992b. Report of the Task Force on Situation Analysis. November. Geneva.

4

Vaccine Demand and Supply

The state of vaccine demand, supply, and innovation on the global level is quite different from that in the United States. Consequently, this chapter examines these trends on a global basis and then explores the domestic conditions of vaccine supply and demand.

GLOBAL DEMAND AND SUPPLY

Demand

The potential size of the worldwide pediatric vaccine market is determined by two factors: the annual worldwide birth cohort (approximately 143 million live births per year) (World Bank, 1993) and the number of vaccines a child receives through adolescence. Eight of the vaccines recommended by the World Health Organization's (WHO's) Expanded Program on Immunization (EPI) should be administered during or shortly after the first year of life (see Appendix G for immunization schedule). According to one estimate, almost 1.5 billion doses of vaccine were used around the world in 1990 (Baudrihaye, 1992) (Table 4-1). Of this amount, North America, Europe, and Japan used just 14 percent of the total, while purchases by the United Nations Children's Fund (UNICEF), the Pan American Health Organization (PAHO), and WHO accounted for approximately 63 percent of the total vaccine used (Baudrihaye, 1992).

Although the number of potential vaccinees in developing countries is

TABLE 4-1 Estimated Worldwide Usage of Vaccines, 1990 (in millions of doses)

Vaccine	North America, Europe, and Japan	UNICEF PAHO, and WHO	Other	Total
BCG	5	160	20	185
DTP	40	219	50	260
Hepatitis B	15		35	50
Influenza	75		10	85
Measles and combined	15	131	30	165
Meningococcal	10	20	30	60
Polio (OPV,IPV)	60	450	190	700
Rabies	1	3	4	8
Total	211	983	358	1,552
Percentage of total	14	63	23	100

SOURCE: Adapted from N. Baudrihaye, European Federation of Pharmaceutical Industries Association, Brussels, 1992; with additional information provided by Akira Homma, PAHO, 1993; John Gilmartin, UNICEF, 1993; Terrel Hill, UNICEF, 1993.

much larger than that in the industrialized world (almost 80 percent of the 143 million live births occur in the developing world), the amount spent on vaccines in the industrialized world greatly exceeds that spent by UNICEF, PAHO, and WHO. The total worldwide value of human vaccines sold in 1992 has been estimated to be as high as $3 billion (Technology Management Group, 1993), of which only $65 million represented UNICEF purchases (John Gilmartin, UNICEF, personal communication, 1993).

Regional Demand

Assessments of country-level demand for vaccines must take into account the size of the target population, estimated extent of immunization coverage, anticipated vaccine wastage, number of scheduled doses, and any special immunization campaigns or strategies that would lead to a surge in demand. Determination of demand for vaccines is more problematic when special, intensive immunization strategies are considered (World Health Organization/Children's Vaccine Initiative, 1992c). For example, the ongoing global campaign to eradicate polio in the Americas has led to increased demand for and, at brief intervals, temporary shortages of polio vaccine (Pan American Health Organization, 1992). In 1992, UNICEF purchased 351 million doses of oral polio vaccine (OPV), which cost $25.6 million including air freight delivery (John Gilmartin, UNICEF, personal communication, 1993; World Health Organization/Children's Vaccine Initiative, 1992b). It is estimated that to duplicate polio eradication efforts elsewhere in the world, the annual purchase of OPV must increase to $87 million (Agency for Cooperation in International Health, 1992).

Vaccine wastage has been identified as another major problem, not only in terms of cost but also in terms of forecasting the demand for vaccine (World Health Organization/Children's Vaccine Initiative, 1992c). Between 1982 and 1992 the demand for EPI vaccines rose 10-fold (Agency for Cooperation in International Health, 1992; UNICEF, 1991b). This kind of growth in demand has forced UNICEF to try to predict the number of doses needed, so that manufacturers will have enough time to increase their production. This has not been an easy task, primarily because the month-to-month variation in demand for a vaccine can vary as much as sevenfold (World Health Organization/Children's Vaccine Initiative, 1992c). Up until 1990, UNICEF's annual forecast of worldwide vaccine demand was fairly accurate. However, in both 1991 and 1992, countries requested substantially less vaccine from UNICEF than estimated (Terrel Hill, UNICEF, personal communication, 1993). The precise reasons for the decreased country demand for UNICEF-supplied vaccine are not fully understood at this time. It is likely, however, that increased local production of vaccines in some countries has led to decreased country-level demand. In addition, improved national census data in many countries may have resulted in a more realistic assessment of vaccine need. Of great concern, however, is that the decreased demand for vaccine may be a result of a slippage in immunization coverage in many countries (Terrel Hill, UNICEF, personal communication, 1993).

Supply

Vaccines are manufactured by both industrialized and developing countries around the world. It is estimated that almost 60 percent of the diphtheria and tetanus toxoids and pertussis vaccine (DTP) currently being used in the world is actually produced in the country that uses it (World Health Organization/Children's Vaccine Initiative, 1992a). The annual production of 500 million doses of EPI vaccines by the People's Republic of China is equivalent to roughly half of all vaccines purchased by UNICEF each year (Agency for Cooperation in International Health, 1992). Currently, OPV is produced or bulk finished in over 25 nations (of which half are considered to be developing countries). (The quality control requirements for the production of OPV differ from those for the finishing of OPV bulk vaccine. For countries to mount full production of OPV, they must maintain expensive monkey colonies, which are needed for neurovirulence testing and must have considerable staff expertise and training. In contrast, finishing a vaccine that has already been fully tested may reduce the need for such large investments in quality control.) Tetanus toxoid is made in almost 40 countries, DTP is manufactured in approximately 30 countries, and measles and BCG (bacillus Calmette-Guérin) vaccines are produced in approximately 20 countries (Agency for Cooperation in International Health, 1992).

The vaccine supply grid developed by Amie Batson and Peter Evans of the World Health Organization (Figure 4-1) depicts the 130 countries that currently produce vaccines according to per capita gross national product and population size. A number of donor agencies are using the grid to evaluate strategies for helping countries buy vaccines, share vaccine production capabilities, or establish production facilities.

Population expansion, more comprehensive immunization, and greatly increased demands for polio vaccine because of global eradication goals have raised questions about the stability of the global vaccine supply (World Health Organization/Children's Vaccine Initiative, 1992a). According to UNICEF, the demand for OPV peaked in 1990 and declined slightly in 1991 and 1992 (Terrel Hill, UNICEF, personal communication, 1993). The largest single user country, India, is expected to become self-sufficient in OPV production in 1993, thereby reducing demand from UNICEF by at least 50 million doses per year (John Gilmartin, UNICEF, personal communication, 1993). UNICEF's ability to procure adequate levels of vaccine into the future is a concern, given rising vaccine prices and competing priorities for increasingly limited resources (UNICEF, 1991a, 1992a); in addition, some donors, such as the Rotary Foundation, have decreased the amount included in their pledges. Preliminary projections of vaccine requirements through 1995 suggest that there may be significant shortfalls in vaccine supply if UNICEF is unable to secure the procurement of EPI vaccines at very low prices into the future. There is also concern that there are now insufficient funds to buy additional EPI vaccines required for such activities as measles control and neonatal tetanus eradication (Agency for Cooperation in International Health, 1991).

At the 1991 International Meeting on Global Vaccine Supply in Kumamoto, Japan, several issues that may affect the future viability of EPI were discussed. Among them were the need to strengthen monetary, logistical, and supply mechanisms for integrating new vaccines into EPI and the need to improve substandard manufacturing capabilities in some countries (Agency for Cooperation in International Health, 1991).

There is mounting concern about the quality of many of the locally produced vaccines used in EPI programs (Hlady et al., 1992; World Health

70

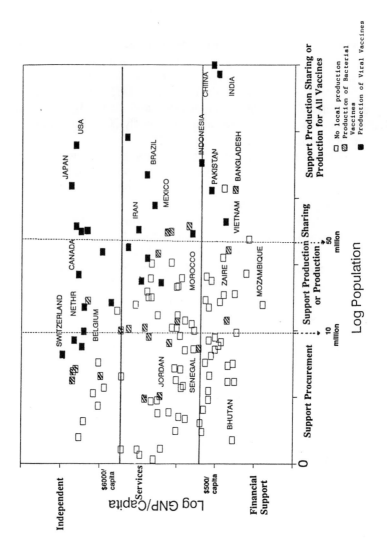

FIGURE 4-1 Vaccine supply grid of countries that produce vaccines according to per capita gross national product (GNP) and population size. SOURCE: Amie Batson and Peter Evans, World Health Organization, 1993.

Organization, 1992). It has been estimated that more than half of the vaccines produced around the world do not meet accepted WHO standards of quality (Lancet, 1992). Many countries lack functioning national control authorities, and as a result, quality control of locally produced vaccines is emerging as a top-priority concern of EPI and the Children's Vaccine Initiative (CVI).

Procurement

UNICEF is the largest single purchaser of vaccine (in doses) for the developing world. The number of doses of EPI vaccines supplied by UNICEF more than doubled in 5 years (Table 4-2). In 1985, UNICEF bought roughly 366 million doses at a cost of approximately $18 million; by 1992, this had increased to 850 million doses at a total cost of some $65 million, including air freight delivery (UNICEF, 1991a, 1992a,b). Polio vaccine and DTP account for the largest number of doses in the UNICEF procurement; this is followed by tetanus toxoid (TT), and BCG and measles vaccine (Table 4-2).

Every 2 years, UNICEF issues a tender for the purchase of vaccines. UNICEF purchases EPI vaccines from all companies that are prequalified to supply vaccine and that submit bids. Companies whose bids are higher than the winning bid are often asked to resubmit an offer. In theory, the lowest bidder receives two-thirds of the UNICEF market, with each successively higher bidder receiving one-third of the remaining market (Peter Evans, Expanded Program on Immunization, World Health Organization, personal communication, 1993). In general, the lowest bidder is unable to

TABLE 4-2 Vaccines Procured by UNICEF, 1985 and 1990

Vaccine	No. of Doses in 1985 (in thousands)	Percent of Total	No. of Doses in 1990 (in thousands)	Percent
BCG	66,296 (4)[a]	18.11	132,004 (5)	13.65
DTP	89,485 (4)	24.45	183,881 (4)	19.01
DT	20,153 (5)	5.51	13,144 (5)	1.36
Measles	36,215 (5)	9.90	86,313 (7)	8.92
OPV	116,772 (5)	1.90	388,510 (6)	40.17
TT	37,049 (4)	10.12	163,400 (6)	16.89
Totals	365,970 (9)		967,254 (11)	

[a] Values in parentheses are number of suppliers.

SOURCE: Data supplied by UNICEF, 1993.

provide UNICEF with two-thirds of the total doses required for any vaccine; therefore, several suppliers provide each vaccine, with preference given to the lowest bidders.

UNICEF has used competitive vaccine bids for many years. From 1985 through 1990, the number of suppliers grew from 9 to 11 (Table 4-2). European vaccine manufacturers supply 90 percent of the vaccines used by UNICEF (this includes Connaught Laboratories, Ltd., [Canada], a subsidiary of Pasteur-Mérieux Sérums et Vaccins) (John Gilmartin, UNICEF, personal communication, 1993). Currently, U.S. vaccine manufacturers are invited to participate in the bidding, but have not made offers since at least 1982. That year, a U.S. vaccine manufacturer was criticized in congressional hearings for selling vaccine to PAHO at prices substantially below those quoted to the U.S. government (U.S. Congress, Senate, 1982). This continues to be a sensitive issue in the United States.

To supply vaccine to UNICEF, a company must request and pay for a WHO-organized evaluation of its manufacturing facilities and the country's national biologics control authority. Several lots of the company's vaccine are then tested at one or more of the WHO's collaborating centers, a process also paid for by the company. Only when the vaccine is determined to meet WHO standards, when the facility is approved, and when the national control authority is determined to be reliable is the company licensed to supply UNICEF with vaccines. UNICEF and WHO do not have the capability to monitor the consistency of vaccine lots produced by manufacturers as is currently done in the United States by the U.S. Food and Drug Administration (see Appendix C).

No manufacturers based in developing countries supplied UNICEF with vaccines in 1990 (Table 4-3). Compared with their international competitors, most vaccine manufacturers in developing countries have several disadvantages. They must frequently import raw materials, often paying substantial import duties on these materials. And because vaccine manufacturing is more capital intensive than labor intensive, the low-cost labor pool in developing countries does not offer any advantages. In fact, some have charged that locally produced vaccines are often more expensive than those procured through UNICEF and PAHO (Baudrihaye, 1992; Vandersmissen, 1992).

Through its procurement system, UNICEF has actively sought to expand the base of suppliers both to ensure a stable vaccine supply and to keep the prices charged for EPI vaccines comparatively low (U.S. Congress, Senate, 1982). (In this regard, UNICEF might be reluctant to purchase a "super" vaccine, such as might result from the CVI, from a single supplier.) UNICEF vaccine prices are a fraction of those commanded elsewhere in the world, including the United States (Table 4-4). Until quite recently, yearly EPI vaccine price increases have barely exceeded inflation. However, in

TABLE 4-3 Companies That Supplied EPI Vaccines to UNICEF, 1990

Company	BCG	DTP	TT	Measles	Polio
Connaught Laboratories, Ltd. (Canada)	X	X	X	X	X
Con Pharma (Canada)			X	X	
Eisai (Japan)				X	
Evans-Medical, Ltd. (United Kingdom)	X			X	
Behringwerke (Hoechst) (Germany)	X	X	X		
Pasteur Mérieux Sérums et Vaccins (France)	X	X	X	X	X
Inter-Export (Yugoslavia)		X	X		
Japan BCG (Japan)	X				
Sclavo (Italy)				X	X
SmithKline Beecham (United Kingdom)				X	X
Swiss Serum Vaccine Institute (Switzerland)		X	X		

SOURCE: Data supplied by UNICEF, January 1993.

TABLE 4-4 UNICEF prices for EPI Vaccine, 1992

Vaccine	No. of Doses	Cost($)/Dose	Cost($)/Series
BCG	1	0.065	0.065
DTP	3	0.0575–0.075	0.173–0.225
Measles	1	0.16	0.16
TT	3–5	0.0325–0.05	0.0975–0.25
OPV	3	0.07–0.085	0.210–0.255
Total	11–13		0.705–0.955

SOURCE: UNICEF Price List, 1992.

1992, vaccine prices increased 23 percent above the 1990 tender price (Steele, 1992). Vaccine manufacturers have indicated that the low prices quoted to UNICEF for EPI vaccines cannot continue indefinitely because the costs of manufacturing vaccines, research and development, and capital investments are all increasing (Mérieux, 1992; Vandersmissen, 1992).

Although some 90 percent of the vaccine purchased by UNICEF and PAHO are made by several of the largest manufacturers, these purchases amount to less than 10 percent of these company's vaccine revenues (Agency for Cooperation in International Health). Indeed, some companies that supply vaccines to UNICEF do so to utilize their excess capacity, and the prices that they charge generally cover the marginal cost of production (Dupuy and Freidel, 1990; Robbins and Freeman, 1988). Because these vaccine purchases have a minimal impact on the total vaccine revenues of those companies that sell vaccine to UNICEF and PAHO, some have suggested that dependence on these international vaccine suppliers puts the global vaccine supply in a precarious position (Agency for Cooperation in International Health, 1992; Institute of Medicine, 1986). Even though a major UNICEF supplier's exit from the vaccine business might have a minor impact on the firm's bottom line, there is concern that it might have a significant negative impact on the supply of high-quality vaccines to the developing world.

Innovation

There are a number of childhood diseases, including malaria and acute respiratory infections, that claim millions of lives annually and for which effective vaccines are not yet available. Unfortunately, the research and development of new and improved vaccines for exclusively developing-country markets by commercial manufacturers is limited. Most public-sector vaccine institutes in Europe do not have the resources or the mandates required to conduct new vaccine development for developing-country markets. The low prices quoted to UNICEF/PAHO cover the marginal costs of production, but they do not appear to provide sufficient market incentives for international vaccine companies to invest in vaccine research and development.

Furthermore, despite a number of successful programs such as the WHO/UNDP Program for Vaccine Development and the UNDP/World Bank/WHO Special Program for Research and Training in Tropical Diseases, there is no significant international or multinational fund dedicated to the early stages of vaccine development and testing of vaccine for use in the developing world.

New and improved vaccines that are developed and manufactured for industrialized-country markets do "trickle down" eventually (sometimes after many years) to some developing countries.   In some cases, vaccines developed by and for the DOD have been introduced into some developing countries on an ad hoc basis by commercial manufacturers.   However, the target groups for these vaccines tend to be adults, not infants and children. This is because the DOD's primary responsibility is to protect young-adult soldiers–not infants and children.   Commercial manufacturers have been reluctant to invest in the costly clinical trials required to demonstrate further vaccine efficacy in infants and young children probably because the returns are likely to be small compared with those from other investment opportunities.   The prices of new vaccines have been beyond the means of most developing countries and such international buyers as UNICEF and PAHO. As a consequence, no new vaccines have been added to the UNICEF procurement scheme since its inception, despite recommendations that hepatitis B vaccine be included in national immunization programs.

DEMAND AND SUPPLY IN THE UNITED STATES

Demand

The pediatric vaccine market in the United States is predictabl↳, limited, and stable. The size of the market is constrained by two factors: the annual birth cohort–approximately 4 million live births per year (World Almanac and Book of Facts, 1992) and the number of vaccines a child receives through adolescence.   Thirteen of the eighteen separate vaccinations recommended by the Advisory Committee on Immunization Practices should be administered during or shortly after the first year of life (see Appendix G for immunization schedule). Three of the remaining four vaccines should be given before age 6 years.

Currently, about 20 million doses of DTP and OPV are distributed each year in the United States (National Vaccine Injury Compensation Trust Fund, 1992).   Prior to the measles epidemic of 1989–1991 and the requirement for a second dose of measles vaccine, approximately 10 million doses of measles-mumps-rubella vaccine (MMR) were distributed each year. In 1990, 19 million doses of MMR were distributed; in 1991, this figure dropped to 16 million (National Vaccine Injury Compensation Trust Fund, 1992).

Over the last decade, the public sector has purchased an increasing share of the vaccines sold in the United States (Table 4-5). Currently, almost half of all vaccines purchased in this country are procured with federal or state funds at contract prices.   The current trend toward public-sector

TABLE 4-5   Publicly Purchased Doses as a Percentage of Net Doses
Distributed in the United States, 1985-1991

Year	DTP	MMR	OPV
1985	15	38	32
1986	29	44	39
1987	45	51	46
1988	33	47	44
1989	35	50	44
1990	40	45	48
1991	43	51	52
1992		54	45

NOTE: Data for 1992 DTP sales to the public are not yet available

SOURCE: Division of Immunization, Centers for Disease Control and Prevention, 1993.

procurement of vaccines is of considerable concern to the large commercial
manufacturers (Douglas, 1992, 1993; Saldarini, 1992, 1993; Williams, 1993).
They argue that sales to the public sector offset those to the private sector,
and increasing public sector procurement will lead to further increases in the
prices charged to private-sector clients (Garnier, 1993). Those involved in
vaccine manufacturing also contend that if the U.S. government emerges as
the sole purchaser of vaccines, company investments in vaccine-related
research and development would likely decline (Douglas, 1992; Katz, 1993;
Saldarini, 1992; Six, 1992). Others (Edelman, 1993; Shalala, 1993) however,
sugges that the effects of any large-scale federal procurement policy on the
U.S. vaccine industry are uncertain—policies on pricing, funding for product
development, and competitive production of vaccines could entice additional
manufacturers to enter this industry (Institute of Medicine, 1986; Shalala,
1993).

Supply

Forty vaccines and toxoids and an additional 10 immune globulins and
antitoxins are licensed and available for use in the United States (see the
box "Vaccines, Toxoids, Immune Globulins, and Antitoxins Available in the
United States, 1993). The current supply of most childhood vaccines is
plentiful in the United States. This is not to say, however, that all children
who should be immunized are or that potential shortages cannot occur.
Nevertheless, the problem of less-than-optimal vaccine coverage in the
United States is due more to problems of access and to the failure of the

Vaccines, Toxoids, Immune Globulins, And Antitoxins Available in the United States, 1993

Licensed Vaccines and Toxoids
Adenovirus vaccine, live oral, type 4
Adenovirus vaccine, live oral, type 7
Anthrax vaccine, adsorbed
BCG (bacillus Calmette Guérin vaccine)
Cholera vaccine
Diphtheria toxoid
Diphtheria toxoid, adsorbed
Diphtheria and tetanus toxoids, adsorbed (TD)
Diphtheria and tetanus toxoids and pertussis vaccine, adsorbed (DTP)
Diphtheria and tetanus toxoids and pertussis vaccine and
   Haemophilus influenzae type b
Diphtheria and tetanus toxoids and acellular pertussis vaccine
   adsorbed (DTaP)
Hepatitis B vaccine, plasma derived
Hepatitis B vaccine, recombinant
Haemophilus type b polysaccaride vaccine
Haemophilus b conjugate vaccine (HbCv)
Influenza virus vaccine
Japanese encephalitis virus vaccine inactivated
Measles virus vaccine live
Measles, mumps and rubella virus vaccine live (MMR)
Measles and mumps virus vaccine live
Measles and rubella virus vaccine live
Meningococcal polysaccaride vaccine A, C, Y, W135 combined
Mumps virus vaccine live
Pertussis vaccine
Pertussis vaccine adsorbed
Poliovirus vaccine inactivated
Polio vaccine live oral, trivalent
Plague vaccine
Pneumococcal vaccine, polyvalent
Rabies vaccine
Rabies vaccine adsorbed
Rubella vaccine
Rubella and mumps virus vaccine live
Smallpox vaccine

Continues

Tetanus toxoid
Tetanus toxoid adsorbed
Tetanus-diptheria (Td)
Typhoid vaccine
Typhoid vaccine, live oral Ty21a
Yellow Fever vaccine

Immune globulins and Antitoxins
Botulism antitoxin
Cytomegalovirus immune globulin intravenous
Diphtheria antitoxin
Hepatitis B immune globulin
Immune globulin
Pertussis immune globulin
Rabies immune globulin
Tetanus antitoxin
Tetanus immune globulin
Vaccinia immune globulin

public health and medical communities to fully immunize all U.S. children than to deficiencies in supply (Cutts et al., 1992; Peter, 1992).

Between 1966 and 1977, half of all commercial vaccine manufacturers in the United States stopped producing and distributing vaccines (U.S. Congress, House, 1986). During the late 1970s and early 1980s, the exodus from the vaccine business continued. Eli Lilly, Pfizer, Glaxo, Wellcome, Dow Chemical, and Merrell-National Laboratories were among those companies that discontinued their vaccine operations or sold off their vaccine components altogether (see Appendix H). The reasons for the exodus during these years are many, but include U.S. Food and Drug Administration requirements for demonstration of vaccine efficacy[1], liability concerns, and poor market returns relative to other product areas. In the United States, the few remaining vaccine manufacturers stayed in the vaccine business as much to meet the public health need (there were no other suppliers for OPV and MMR) as out of corporate commitment to their products.

Although 18 companies and two states are licensed to manufacture selected vaccines for the U.S. market, only a handful of companies supply pediatric vaccines. The supply of two of the vaccines, MMR and OPV, is dependent on sole-source suppliers (U.S. Department of Health and Human Services, 1991). Reliance on such a small number of companies for the production of U.S. pediatric vaccines has not been without problems

(Institute of Medicine, 1985; U.S. Congress, House, 1986). A series of unfortunate events in 1984 and early 1985 led to a shortage of DTP in the United States: two private-sector manufacturers withdrew from the market because of liability concerns (among other reasons), and a third manufacturer experienced some production problems. State manufacturers of DTP could not meet the demand, and the Centers for Disease Control and Prevention (CDC) had to issue a revised immunization schedule that urged physicians to delay giving some DTP booster shots until more vaccine became available (U.S. Congress, House, 1986). The fragility of the nation's vaccine supply had been demonstrated.

In 1983, Congress appropriated funds to the CDC to ensure that a 6-month stockpile of critical vaccines be maintained at all times as a solution to a temporary shortage of vaccine. Although a 6-month stockpile would compensate for short-term interruptions in supply, it is unlikely that U.S. immunization efforts could be sustained if a sole producer of a vaccine were to halt the production and distribution of a needed product. It takes considerably more than 6 months to retrofit an existing production facility to make a new vaccine and longer still to construct a facility from the ground up (George Siber, Massachusetts Department of Public Health, personal communication, 1993).

Pricing

In the United States, commercial manufacturers list two pri   lor a vaccine: a contract price, which is negotiated on an annual basis w...i the CDC, and a catalog price, which sets vaccine prices for private-sector clients, such as hospitals, health maintenance organizations, pharmacies, and physicians. As can be seen in Table 4-6, the catalog price for each

TABLE 4-6 Cost and Price (including Excise Tax) of the Basic Series of Childhood Vaccines in the United States, as of March 31, 1993

| Vaccine | Price ($) | | No. of | Cost ($) | |
	Contract	Catalog	Doses	Public Sector	Private Sector
DTaP	11.01	16.33	2	22.02	32.66
DTP	5.99	10.04	3	17.97	30.12
Hib-CV	5.37	15.13	4	21.48	60.52
MMR	15.33	25.29	2	30.66	50.58
OPV	2.16	10.43	4	8.64	41.72
Hepatitis B	6.91	10.71	3	20.73	32.12
Total			18	121.50	247.72

SOURCE: Division of Immunization, Centers for Disease Control and Prevention, 1993.

childhood vaccine is higher than the contract price. The total public-sector cost of the required pediatric vaccines in 1993 is $122, while the cost to private-sector clients is more than double that ($248). Although there are differences in the terms and conditions of vaccine sales to the public and private sectors (companies bear the cost of distributing catalog-priced vaccines and buy back unused doses), sales to the private sector are said to offset those to the public sector. As the percentage of doses procured by the public sector has increased over time, vaccine prices in the private sector have risen substantially.

Excluding the cost of vaccine, the charges associated with administering the complete series of pediatric vaccines may run from as little as $25 at a public health clinic to more than $200 at a private physician's office (Freeman et al., 1993). Thus, the total amount, including vaccine, needed to fully immunize a child in the United States ranges from almost $147 in the public sector to more than $448 in the private sector.

In 1988, in an effort to compensate for adverse events from government-mandated vaccines as well as to offset vaccine manufacturers' liability concerns, an excise tax was added to the price of each of the government-mandated childhood vaccines. Until recently, the taxes–$4.56 per dose of DTP, $4.44 per dose of MMR, and $0.29 per dose of OPV–were paid into a special trust fund that was used to pay the claims of those with vaccine-related injuries. The law establishing the National Vaccine Injury Compensation Program mandated that the excise taxes be collected until 1992, at which point the program was to be reassessed. A provision to extend the National Vaccine Injury Compensation Program was included as part of a larger congressional bill, which was subsequently vetoed for reasons unrelated to the compensation program. Because there was no further congressional action to extend the collection of excise taxes, the Secretary of the Treasury, in accordance with the law, revoked the excise tax in January 1993. This situation has caused some confusion, but is expected to be resolved shortly by Congress. (See Appendix B for a discussion of the National Vaccine Injury Compensation Program.)

The list price for each of the major government-mandated childhood vaccines in both the public and private sectors has increased substantially since 1977 (see Table 4-7). Tables 4-8 and 4-9 show federal contract and private catalog prices, respectively, in constant dollars for OPV, DTP, and MMR for the period 1977–1992. For comparison, the last three columns in Tables 4-8 and 4-9 present the indices used to track changes in the prices of various goods. The first, the Consumer Price Index (CPI), reflects the price rise of a general "basket" of consumer goods; the second, the Pharmaceutical Producer Price Index (PPPI), reflects price changes in ethical pharmaceuticals. Prices in both indices are standardized to the base year of 1983.

TABLE 4-7 Vaccine Prices (in dollars) in the United States from 1977–February 1993

Year	DTP		OPV		MMR		Hib-CV	
	CP	FC	CP	FC	CP	FC	CP	FC
1977	0.19	0.15[a]	1.00	0.30	6.01	2.42	NA	NA
1978	0.22	0.15[a]	1.15	0.31	6.16	2.35	NA	NA
1979	0.25	0.15[a]	1.27	0.33	6.81	2.62	NA	NA
1980	0.30	0.15[a]	1.60	0.35	7.24	2.71	NA	NA
1981	0.33	0.15[a]	2.10	0.40	9.32	3.12	NA	NA
1982	0.37	0.15[a]	2.75	0.48	10.44	4.02	NA	NA
1983	0.45	0.42[a]	3.56	0.58	11.30	4.70	NA	NA
1984	0.99	0.65[a]	4.60	0.73	12.08	5.40	NA	NA
1985	2.80	2.21	6.15	0.80	13.53	6.85	NA	NA
1986	11.40	3.01	8.67	1.56	15.15	8.47	NA	NA
1987	8.92	7.69	8.07	1.36	17.88	10.67	NA	NA
1988	11.03	8.46[b]	8.07	1.36	24.11	16.18	13.75	11.00
1989	10.65	7.96	9.45	1.92	24.11	16.18	13.75	6.00
1990	10.65	6.91	9.74	1.92	24.07	14.71	14.55	5.20
1991	9.97	6.25	9.45	2.00	25.29	15.33	14.55	5.16[c]
1992	9.97	6.25	9.91	2.09	25.29	15.30	14.55	5.16[c]
1993	10.04	5.99	10.43	2.16	25.29	15.33	15.13	5.37

NOTE: CP, Catalog Price; FC, Federal contract Price; NA, vaccine not licensed. From 1988 to 1992, prices include federal excise tax for the Vaccine Injury Compensation Program. Excise taxes are set at $4.56 per dose of DTP, $4.44 per dose of MMR, and $0.29 per dose of OPV.

[a] No federal contract. The price represents the average price charged to the states.

[b] Federal contract price was $9.62 for a portion of 1988.

[c] Merck federal contract price was $8.25 for use among Native American populations.

SOURCE: Division of Immunization, Centers for Disease Control and Prevention, 1993.

It is worth noting that through the early 1980s, the prices of OPV and DTP were quite low, an indication, the committee believes, that manfacturers were treating vaccines much like generic products that cost little to produce, that had high-volume sales, and that had low profit margins. Vaccines appear to have been priced to cover their marginal costs of production. Indeed, companies marketed DTP at roughly $0.15 a dose and OPV at $0.30 a dose to the federal goverment into the early 1980s.

Beginning in the early 1980s and continuing to the present, vaccine prices have risen substantially. Over the 15-year period from 1977 to 1991, the cumulative increases (in 1993 dollars and excluding the excise tax) in the contract and catalog prices for DTP were $1.55 (1,033 percent increase) and $5.22 (2,847 percent increase) respectively. The cumulative increase in the price of OPV from 1977 through 1992 was $8.62, or 500 percent for the contract price of vaccine, and $1.50, or 862 percent, for the catalog price of vaccine. From 1977 through 1992, the contract price for MMR increased by $8.47, or 350 percent, wheras the catalog price rose by $14.84, or 247 percent. During this same period, the CPI rose 122 percent and the PPPI jumped 232 percent.

The rate of price increases in the market for DTP, MMR, and OPV has outstripped the rise in prices for the economy as a whole and for ethical pharmaceuticals. Those companies that remained in the vaccine business after the exodus in the 1970s appear now to be treating vaccines much like other pharmaceutical products with a corresponding investment in new facilities and in research and development and with an anticipation of returns.

Vaccine Innovation

The pharmaceutical industry has often been described as a high-risk, high-profit enterprise that is dependent upon the development and marketing of novel products (di Masi et al., 1991; Grabowski and Vernon, 1990; Lasagna, 1992; Office of Technology Assessment, 1991). Most established pharmaceutical firms have viewed the vaccine business as unpromising, characterized by undifferentiated product lines, a high risk of product liability, a few large high-volume, low-price purchasers, and poor patent protection (DeBrock, 1983; Institute of Medicine, 1985, 1986; Nicholas Mellors, Merlin, personal communication, 1993; Vandersmissen, 1992). The exodus of companies from the vaccine business in the 1960s through 1970s (see Appendix H), the relatively low expenditures on research and development into the 1980s (Table 4-10), and the small proportion (less than 5 percent) of vaccine Product License Applications (PLAs) as a total of all PLAs filed at the Center for Biologics and Evaluation Research from 1987 to 1991 would appear at the outset to confirm this assessment.

The pharmaceutical industry devotes a relatively small share of its research and development expenditures to biologics, a category that includes vaccines (Table 4-10). This is hardly surprising since vaccine sales account for less than 5 percent of most diversified companies' total sales (Agency for Cooperation in International Health, 1991; American Cyanamid, 1991; Institute of Medicine, 1992; Merck & Co., Inc., 1991b). Although spending in real terms (as reported to the Pharmaceutical Manufacturers Association) on pharmaceutical and biologics R&D has increased over time, the pattern of investment in biologics R&D has, until very recently, been one of decline. Spending on biologics research fell from 4 percent of the total in 1973 to a little more than 2 percent in 1983. By 1988, spending on biologics R&D had returned to the 1973 level (in relative terms), and it has increased every

TABLE 4-8 Federal Contract Prices for Vaccines in "Current" Dollars

Year	Price of OPV ($)	PI	Price of MMR ($)	PI	Price of DTP ($)	Price Indices CPI	PPPI
1977	0.30	51	2.42	51	0.15	61	59
1978	0.31	54	2.35	50	0.15	65	62
1979	0.33	57	2.62	56	0.15	73	67
1980	0.35	61	2.71	58	0.15	82	73
1981	0.40	68	3.12	66	0.15	91	81
1982	0.48	82	4.02	86	0.15	97	90
1983	0.58	100	4.70	100	0.42	100	100
1984	0.73	125	5.40	115	0.65	104	109
1985	0.80	138	6.85	146	2.21	108	119
1986	1.56	268	8.47	180	3.01	110	130
1987	1.36	234	10.67	227	7.69	114	141
1988	1.07	184	11.74	250	3.90	118	152
1989	1.63	280	11.74	250	3.40	124	166
1990	1.63	280	10.27	219	2.35	131	181
1991	1.71	294	10.89	232	1.70	136	196
1992	1.80	310	10.89	232	1.70	140	208

NOTE: Prices are indexed at a base year of 1983. PI, price index. Prices exclude the excise taxes for the Vaccine Injury Compensation Program that were in effect from 1988 to January 1993.

SOURCE: Bureau of Labor Statistics, U.S. Department of Labor; Centers for Disease Control.

TABLE 4-9 Private Catalog Prices for Vaccines in "Current" Dollars

Year	Price of OPV ($)	PI	Price of MMR ($)	PI	Price of DTP ($)	Price Indices CPI	Price Indices PPPI
1977	1.00	28	6.01	53	0.19	61	59
1978	1.15	32	6.16	55	0.22	65	62
1979	1.27	36	6.81	60	0.25	73	67
1980	1.60	45	7.24	64	0.30	82	73
1981	2.10	59	9.32	82	0.33	91	81
1982	2.75	77	10.44	92	0.37	97	90
1983	3.56	100	11.30	100	0.45	100	100
1984	4.60	129	12.08	107	0.99	104	109
1985	6.15	173	13.53	120	2.80	108	119
1986	8.67	244	15.15	134	11.40	110	130
1987	8.07	227	17.88	158	8.92	114	141
1988	7.78	219	19.67	174	6.47	118	152
1989	9.16	257	19.67	174	6.09	124	166
1990	9.45	265	19.63	174	6.09	131	181
1991	9.16	257	20.85	185	5.41	136	196
1992	9.62	270	20.85	185	5.41	140	208

NOTE: Prices are indexed at a base year of 1983. PI, price index. Prices exclude the excise taxes for the Vaccine Injury Compensation Program that were in effect from 1988 to January 1993.

SOURCE: Bureau of Labor Statistics, U.S. Department of Labor; Centers for Disease Control.

year since then. Of more relevance, however, is spending on vaccine R&D as a percentage of total vaccine sales. This percentage decreased substantially from 1976 to 1982 (Table 4-10). Although recent data on vaccine R&D as a percentage of vaccine sales are unreported and unavailable, it is likely that investment in R&D has increased to 12–15 percent of sales, which is similar to that for the overall pharmaceutical industry (Business Week, 1992; Financial Times, 1993).

The total number of Investigational New Drug (IND) applications submitted to the Center for Biologics Evaluation and Research of the U.S. Food and Drug Administration (FDA) has increased dramatically, from 66 in 1980 to just under 558 in 1992 (Zoon and Beatrice, 1993). Almost half of the IND applications filed since the mid-1980s are for biologic products produced by using biotechnology (Figure 4-2). Although almost four times as many IND applications were submitted for therapeutics than for vaccines in 1992 (Figure 4-3), there has been a notable increase in the number of vaccine IND applications filed in the last several years. From 1983 through 1989, an average of 32 vaccine IND applications were filed each year. In 1990, 67 vaccine IND applications were filed; in 1992, 81 were filed (Zoon and Beatrice, 1993). Thus, it appears that the relatively low number of PLAs filed during the late 1980s and early 1990s reflects both the lengthy development timeline of vaccines and the time-consuming FDA licensure process. Many more vaccine-related PLAs can be expected in the future.

There are other signs that vaccines are becoming more important relative to other operations of pharmaceutical companies. For example, Merck & Co., Inc., created the Merck Vaccine Division in 1991, and Lederle-Praxis Biologicals was made a full business unit of American Cyanamid in 1992. Corporate-level reorganization has also translated into major capital investments for some companies. Indeed, Merck & Co., Inc., is investing $150 million in the construction of a biotechnology facility for vaccines in Pennsylvania (Douglas, 1993).

Established pharmaceutical firms with vaccine interests are also actively pursuing promising technologies developed by various biotechnology companies by either licensing the technology or simply buying the company outright (Sugawara, 1992). In 1989, Lederle Laboratories, a unit of the American Cyanamid Corporation, acquired Praxis Biologics, a biotechnology company that had developed a conjugate *Haemophilus influenzae* type b conjugate vaccine (Hib-CV). Merck & Co., Inc., has entered into a variety of strategic alliances with a variety of companies, including MedImmune, Inc., a biotechnology firm involved in vaccine development (MedImmune, 1991; Merck & Co., Inc., 1991a). By the end of 1992, there were over 75

TABLE 4-10 R&D Expenditures and Sales of All U.S. Pharmaceuticals and of the Biologics Component

| Year | R&D Expenditures | | | Sales | | | Total R&D/ Total Sales (percent) | Biologics R&D/ Biologics Sales (percent) |
	Pharmaceuticals (millions of $)	Biologics (millions of $)	Biologics Component (percent)	Pharmaceuticals (millions of $)	Biologics (millions of $)	Biologics Component (percent)		
1973	644	25.7	4.0	5,122	138.3	2.7	12.57	18.58
1974	726	32.7	4.5	5,657	152.7	2.7	12.83	21.41
1975	829	24.9	3.0	6,412	160.3	2.5	12.92	15.53
1976	903	28.0	3.1	7,117	121.0	1.7	12.69	23.14
1977	984	30.5	3.1	7,705	169.5	2.2	12.77	17.99
1978	1,089	34.9	3.2	8,424	235.9	2.8	12.93	14.79
1979	1,243	31.0	2.5	9,240	240.2	2.6	13.45	12.91
1980	1,455	45.1	3.1	11,091	244.0	2.2	13.12	18.48
1981	1,765	42.3	2.4	13,000	468.0	3.6	13.58	9.04
1982	2,158	49.6	2.3	15,394	538.8	3.5	14.02	9.21
1983	2,538	53.3	2.1	16,565			15.32	
1984	2,843							
1985	3,234	84.1	2.6	21,205			15.25	
1986	3,721	85.6	2.3	24,032			15.48	
1987	4,342	121.6	2.8	27,019			16.07	
1988	5,051	207.1	4.1	29,692			17.01	
1989	5,824	273.7	4.7	33,469			17.40	
1990	6,446							
1991	7,276							

NOTE: All data are for members of the Pharmaceutical Manufacturers Association. R&D expenditures are for company-financed R&D for ethical pharmaceuticals and biologics for human use. Biologics include bacterial and viral vaccines, antigens, antitoxins, toxoids, and allogenic extracts as well as sera, plasma, and other blood derivatives for human use.
[a] Sales of biologics are unavailable for 1983 to present.

SOURCE: PMA Survey of Members, Annual Survey Report; Timothy Brogan, personal communication, Pharmaceutical Manufacturers Association, 1992.

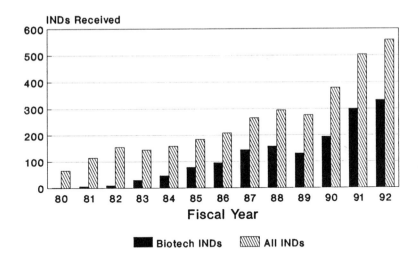

FIGURE 4-2 CBER biotech INDs received, compared to total. SOURCE: Application Review and Policy, Therapeutics Research and Review, Center for Biologics Evaluation and Research, U.S. Food and Drug Administration.

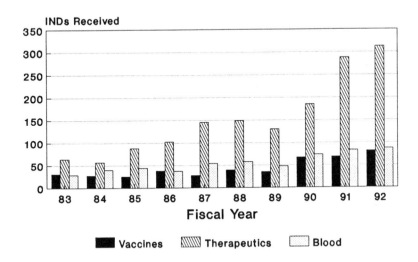

FIGURE 4-3 CBER INDs received, by category. SOURCE: Application Review and Policy, Therapeutics Research and Review, Center for Biologics Evaluation and Research, U.S. Food and Drug Administration.

biotechnology companies worldwide (most of them in the United States) conducting vaccine-related R&D (Oryx Press, 1992).

There is also considerable international activity in the area of vaccine innovation. A number of U.S. companies are entering into cross-licensing arrangements with European and Japanese partners, and European companies are acquiring firms that have access to the U.S. market. In 1989, Institut Mérieux acquired Connaught Laboratories, Inc., and Merck and Company entered into a product development and licensing agreement with Pasteur Mérieux Sérums et Vaccins in 1993. Chiron, a U.S. biotechnology firm, joined with Ciba-Geigy, an established Swiss-based pharmaceutical firm, to purchase the financially troubled Sclavo, an Italian manufacturer of vaccines in 1990 (Chiron Corporation, 1991). A number of biotechnology companies involved in vaccine-related R&D have entered into strategic alliances with Japanese companies (National Research Council, 1992).

A review of the vaccines licensed for use in the United States since 1986 shows that approximately half are new (Table 4-11). This is markedly different from the situation just 10 years ago. A majority of the vaccines licensed in the 1970s were improvements of old vaccines (Institute of Medicine, 1985). A recently licensed vaccine against typhoid resembles a product, in some respects, that might be used in the CVI, but it was developed in part by and for the DOD.

The current vaccine development process in the United States, from basic research through to the production, distribution, and marketing of vaccine products, although poorly integrated, does lead to the development and production of new vaccines for the domestic market, primarily because vaccine manufacturers perceive there to be adequate returns on their investment. An indication of the level of vaccine innovation is the sheer number of vaccines in various stages of development in the United States (Table 4-12). As can be seen, however, few of the vaccines currently being developed by established vaccine manufacturers are for exclusive use in the developing world, simply because such vaccines are perceived to be without sufficient returns on investment. As noted earlier, some vaccines developed by or for the DOD have been introduced into some developing countries on an ad hoc basis by commercial manufacturers. A few small biotechnology firms are working on vaccines of potential benefit to the developing world. As discussed in Chapter 3 and later in this report, few of these companies have the capacity to take a vaccine through to licensure and full-scale manufacture. Most of the development-stage companies working on vaccines of relevance to the developing world do so as part of cooperative research and development agreements (CRADAs) with the U.S. Department of Defense, and to a lesser extent, with the National Institute of Allergy and Infectious Diseases. At this time, the Walter Reed Army Institute of Research has almost 40 CRADAs with private-sector firms, the vast majority of which are development-stage biotechnology companies based in the United States (LTC Willis A. Reid, Chief, Office of Research and Technology Applications, Walter Reed Army Institute of Research, personal communication, 1993).

By all accounts, the worldwide vaccine industry appears to be entering a new era of activity and innovation. In the United States, commercial vaccine manufacturers and biotechnology firms are pursuing the development of innovative vaccine products targeted to the industrialized-world market. The development and manufacture of vaccines for exclusively developing-world markets are not attractive investments for either commercial vaccine manufacturers or biotechnology firms because they are unlikely to offer adequate returns on investments under current market arrangements.

TABLE 4-11   Vaccines Licensed for Use in the United States Since 1986

Vaccine and Company	Review Time (months)	FDA Approval	Characteristics
BCG live Connaught Laboratories, Inc.	18.1	05/1990	New approval of an old vaccine for limited indication (treatment of carcinoma-in-situ of the urinary bladder
BCG vaccine Organon Teknika Corporation	29.5	08/1990	New approval of old vaccine (also indicated for the treatment of carcinoma-in-situ of the urinary bladder
Diphtheria and tetanus toxoids and acellular pertussis vaccine, adsorbed (DTaP) Lederle-Praxis Biologicals	51.5	12/1991	New acellular pertussis component; shared manufacture with Takeda Chemical Industries, Ltd.
Diphtheria and tetanus toxoids and acellular pertussis vaccine, adsorbed (DTaP) Connaught Laboratories, Inc.	27.1	08/1992	New acellular component; shared manufacture with Biken (Research Foundation of Osaka University)
Diphtheria and tetanus toxoids and pertussis vaccine, adsorbed and *Haemophilus influenzae* type b conjugate Lederle-Praxis Biologicals	14.9	03/1993	New vaccine
Haemophilus influenzae type b meningococcal outer membrane conjugate vaccine Merck & Co., Inc.	24.9	12/1989	New vaccine (18–60 months)
Haemophilus influenzae type b meningococcal outer membrane conjugate vaccine Merck & Co., Inc.	4.1	12/1990	Infant indication
Haemophilus influenzae type b conjugate vaccine (tetanus toxoid conjugate) Pasteur Mérieux Sérums et Vaccins	27.8	03/1993	New vaccine
Haemophilus influenzae type b and diphtheria CRM 197 protein conjugate vaccine Praxis Biologics, Inc.	22.5	12/1988	New vaccine (18–60 months)
Haemophilus influenzae type b conjugate vaccine Praxis Biologics, Inc.	6.9	10/1990	Infant indication

TABLE 4-11 *Continued*

Vaccine and Company	Review Time (months)	FDA Approval	Characteristics
Haemophilus influenzae type b conjugate (diphtheria toxoid conjugate) Connaught Laboratories, Inc.	55.4	12/1987	New vaccine (18–60 months)
Hepatitis B vaccine, recombinant Merck & Co., Inc.	18.0	07/1986	New vaccine
Hepatitis B vaccine, recombinant SmithKline Beecham	20.8	08/1989	Independent introduction
Influenza virus vaccine Evans Medical, Ltd.	17.3	08/1988	New introduction of old vaccine
Japanese encephalitis virus, inactivated Research Foundation of Osaka University Connaught Laboratories, Inc.	30.8	12/1992	New vaccine
Poliovirus vaccine, inactivated Connaught Laboratories, Inc.	16.1	11/1987	Enhanced poliovirus vaccine
Poliovirus vaccine, inactivated Pasteur Mérieux Sérums et Vaccins	93.3	12/1990	Independent introduction
Rabies vaccine, adsorbed Michigan Department of Public Health	93.3	03/1988	Independent introduction
Rabies vaccine Connaught Laboratories, Inc.	42.4	12/1991	Independent introduction
Typhoid vaccine, live oral (Ty-21a) Swiss Serum & Vaccine Institute, Berne	92.5	12/1989	New vaccine

SOURCES: New Drug Approvals in 1991, Pharmaceutical Manufacturers Association, January 1992; New Drug Approvals in 1990, Pharmaceutical Manufacturers Association, January 1991; New Drug Approvals in 1989, Pharmaceutical Manufacturers Association, January 1990; Biotechnology Medicines, Pharmaceutical Manufacturers Association, 1990; Douglas Reynolds, Connaught Laboratories, Swiftwater, Pennsylvania, October 1992; Carolyn Hardegree, Center for Biologics Evaluation and Research, U.S. Food and Drug Administration.

TABLE 4-12   Selected Vaccines in Development

Product and Company	U.S. Development Status
Adenohepatitis B virus vaccine Wyeth-Ayerst	Phase I
Acellular pertussis vaccine Massachusetts Department of Public Health	Phase I/II
Acellular pertussis component Michigan Department of Public Health	Phase I

Diphtheria and tetanus toxoids and
  acellular pertussis vaccine, adsorbed
  Lederle-Praxis Biologicals
	Phase III (infant efficacy study)

Diphtheria and tetanus toxoids and
  acellular pertussis vaccine, adsorbed
  North American Vaccine
	Phase III

Diphtheria and tetanus toxoids and
  accellular pertussis vaccine, adsorbed
  and inactivated polio vaccine
  North American Vaccine
	Phase III

Tetrammune™ Diphtheria and tetanus toxoids
  and pertussis vaccine, adsorbed, and
  Haemophilus influenzae type b vaccine
  Lederle-Praxis Biologicals
	PLA submitted (recommended
	  for approval by FDA advisory
	  committee, ages 2 months up
	  to 7th birthday)

Diptheria and tetanus toxoids and acellular
  pertussis vaccine, adsorbed, and
  Haemophilus influenzae type b
  conjugate vaccine
  Lederle-Praxis Biologicals
	Phase II (for booster dose at
	  15–18 months of age or when
	  both vaccines recommended to
	  be given simultaneouly)

Propedia™ Diphtheria and tetanus toxoids
  and pertussis vaccine, adsorbed and
  Haemophilus influenzae type b vaccine
  (diphtheria toxoid conjugate)
  Connaught Laboratories, Inc.
	PLA submitted (for 15–60 months
	  of age as final booster dose in Hib
	  series or as a single dose primary
	  immunization at 15–60 months of
	  age)

ActHIB™ + DTP; Diptheria and tetanus toxoids
  ActHIB and pertussis vaccine, adsorbed,
  reconstituting *Haemophilus influenzae*
  type b conjugate vaccine (tetanus
  protein conjugate)
  Connaught Laboratories, Inc./Pasteur
  Mérieux Sérums et Vaccins
	Submitted as part of PLA for
	  alone (for 2–60 months of age)

ActHIB™ + DTaP; Diptheria and tetanus toxoids
  and acellular pertussis vaccine, adsorbed,
  reconstituting *Haemophilus influenzae*
  type b conjugate vaccine (tetanus protein
  conjugate)
  Connaught Laboratories, Inc./Pasteur
  Mérieux Sérums et Vaccins
	Phase II for 15–60 months of age

TABLE 4-12 *Continued*

Product and Company	Development Status
Diphtheria and tetanus toxoids and pertussis vaccine, *Haemophilus influenzae* type b, hepatitis B vaccine Merck & Co., Inc./Connaught Laboratories, Inc.	Phase I (by summer of 1993)
Diphtheria and tetanus toxoids and pertussis vaccine, *Haemophilus influenzae* type b, hepatitis B vaccine and inactivated polio vaccine Merck & Co., Inc./Connaught Laboratories, Inc.	Phase I (by summer of 1993)

Diphtheria and tetanus toxoids and pertussis vaccine, hepatitis B and *Haemophilus influenzae* type b conjugate vaccine
    Michigan Department of Public Health/
    SmithKline Beecham
	Pre-clinical studies completed; preparing IND submissions

Diphtheria and tetanus toxoids and acellular pertussis vaccine and hepatitis B vaccine and *Haemophilus influenzae* type b conjugate vaccine
    Michigan Department of Public Health/
    SmithKline Beecham
	Pre-clinical studies completed; preparing IND submissions

Diptheria and tetanus toxoids and pertussis vaccine, adsorbed, and poliovirus vaccine, inactivated Connaught Laboratories, Inc./Pasteur Mérieux Sérums et Vaccins	PLA submitted
ActHIB™ *Haemophilus influenzae* type b conjugate vaccine (tetanus protein conjugate) Connaught Laboratories, Inc./Pasteur Mérieux Sérums et Vaccins	PLA submitted
Haemophilus influenzae type b conjugate vaccine Massachusetts Department of Public Health	Phase III
Haemophilus influenzae type b conjugate vaccine, hepatitis B vaccine Merck & Co., Inc.	Phase III
VAQTA™ hepatitis A vaccine Merck & Co., Inc.	Phase III
Hepatitis B vaccine Connaught Laboratories, Inc.	Phase II
Hepatitis B vaccine Amgen/Johnson & Johnson	Phase III
Herpes vaccine Lederle-Praxis Biologicals	Phase I (adults)
Pryme™ lyme disease vaccine (recombinant OspA lipoprotein for Lyme borreliosis) Connaught Laboratories, Inc.	Phase I

Continues

TABLE 4-12 *Continued*

Product and Company	Development Status
Lyme disease vaccine (recombinant OspA lipoprotein for Lyme borreliosis) SmithKline Beecham	Phase I (by summer of 1993)
M-M-R®$_{II}$ measles, mumps, rubella, and varicella Merck & Co., Inc.	Phase III
Measles, mumps, rubella virus vaccine, live Connaught Laboratories, Inc./Pasteur Mérieux Sérums et Vaccins	Project currently inactive
Meningococcal group B vaccine (outer membrane protein) Connaught Laboratories, Inc.	Phase III for 2 years of age and older
Pneumococcal conjugate vaccine (streptococcal conjugate vaccine, diphtheria toxoid and tetanus protein conjugates for otitis media and pneumonia) Connaught Laboratories, Inc./Pasteur Mérieux Sérums et Vaccins	Phase I
Pneumococcal conjugate vaccine, streptococcal pneumonia vaccine, enhanced Lederle-Praxis Biologicals	Phase I/II
Pneumococcal conjugate vaccine Merck & Co., Inc.	Phase II
Respiratory syncytial virus vaccine Lederle-Praxis Biologicals	Phase I/II
Rhesus rotavirus vaccine Wyeth-Ayerst	Phase III
Rhesus rotavirus vaccine Merck & Co., Inc.	Phase II
Sabin IPV inactivated Sabin polio vaccine Lederle-Praxis Biologicals	Phase III (age 2 months and up)
Salmonella, live attenuated Lederle-Praxis Biologicals	Phase I
Streptococcal group B vaccine North American Vaccine	Phase I
Varivax® varicella vaccine Merck & Co., Inc.	PLA submitted

SOURCES: Pharmaceutical Manufacturers Association. 1990. New Medicines in Development for Children. Washington, D.C.; Pharmaceutical Manufacturers Association. 1990. Biotechnology Medicines. Washington, D.C.; Douglas Reynolds, Connaught Laboratories, Inc., October 1992; Glenna Crooks and Ronald B. Ellis, Merck & Co., Inc., May 1993; Jane Scott, Lederle-Praxis Biologicals, February 1993; George Siber, Massachusetts Biologic Laboratories, June 1993; Robert Meyers, Michigan Department of Public Health, May 1993; Dan Soland, SmithKline Beecham, June 1993.

NOTE

1. When the Division of Biologics (DBS) became a part of the Food and Drug Administration in 1972, the Commissioner of Food and Drugs appointed vaccine advisory panels to evaluate the safety and effectiveness of biological products licensed prior to 1972 (USC § 601.22, 21 CFR Ch.1). Several vaccines were found not to be safe and/or effective or in many other cases the manufacturers did not submit the required information for evaluation of their vaccines, but requested the FDA to revoke the licenses without prejudice.

REFERENCES

Agency for Cooperation in International Health. 1991. Report of the International Meeting on Global Vaccine Supply, May 23–26, Kumamoto, Japan.

Agency for Cooperation in International Health. 1992. Report of the Second International Meeting on Global Vaccine Supply, August 3–5, Tokyo, Japan.

American Cyanamid. 1991. Form 10-K. Washington, D.C: Securities and Exchange Commission.

Baudrihaye N. 1992. European vaccine manufacturers: Present status and future trends. Vaccine 10:893–5.

Business Week. 1992. R&D Scoreboard: On a clear day you can see progress. June 29. New York: McGraw Hill, Inc.

Chiron Corporation. 1991. Annual Report. Emeryville, California.

Cutts FT, Bernier RH, Orenstein WA. 1992. Causes of low preschool immunization coverage in the United States. Annual Review of Public Health 13:385–398.

DeBrock, LM. 1983. The domestic vaccine industry: The economic framework. Paper presented at the Institute of Medicine Conference on Barriers to Vaccine Innovation, November 28–29, Washington, D.C.

Di Masi J, Hansen RW, Grabowski HG, Lasagna L. 1991. Cost of innovation in the pharmaceutical industry. Journal of Health Economics 10:107–142.

Douglas GR. 1993. Testimony before the Subcommittee on Access to Immunization Services, National Vaccine Advisory Committee. A Public Hearing on the Economic and Commercial Underpinning of Vaccine Supply, February 24, Bethesda, Maryland.

Douglas GR. 1992. Testimony before the Senate Subcommittee on Appropriations. Childhood vaccine research and development Issues. April 8. Washington, D.C.

Dupuy JM Freidel L. 1990. Lag between discovery and producing of new vaccines for the developing world. Lancet 336:733–734.

Edelman, MW. 1993. Testimony of the Children's Defense Fund. Senate Labor and Human Resources Committee and the House Subcommittee on Health and Environment. April 21. Washington, D.C.

Financial Times. 1993. Pharmaceuticals: Research and Development. April 22. Pp. 1-6.

Freeman P, Johnson K, Babcock J. 1993. A health challenge for the states: Achieving full benefit of childhood immunization. Occasional paper. February. The John W. McCormack Institute of Public Affairs, University of Massachusetts at Boston.

Garnier, JP. 1993. Testimony before the Senate Committee on Labor and Human Resources and the House Subcommittee on Health and the Environment. April 21, 1993. Washington, D.C.

Grabowski H Vernon J. 1990. A new look at the returns and risks to pharmaceutical R&D. Management Science 36:804–821.

Hlady GW, Bennett JV, Samadi AR, Begum J, Hafez A, Tarafdar AI, Boring JR. 1992. Neonatal tetanus in rural Bangladesh: Risk factors and toxoid efficacy. American Journal of Public Health 82:1365–1369.

Hoover's Handbook of American Business. 1992. Emeryville, California: The Reference Press, Inc.

Institut Mérieux International. 1990. Annual Report. Lyon, France.

Institute of Medicine. 1985. Vaccine Supply and Innovation. Washington, D.C.: National Academy Press.

Institute of Medicine. 1986. Proceedings of a Workshop on Vaccine Supply and Innovation. Report for the Subcommittee on Oversight and Investigations, Committee on Energy and Commerce. U.S. Congress, House. August. Washington, D.C.

Institute of Medicine. 1992. Proceedings from Working Groups on The Children's Vaccine Initiative: Planning Alternative Strategies Towards Full U.S. Participation. June. Washington, D.C.

Katz S. 1993. Could the Childhood Vaccine Act Be Bad? Letter to the Editor. Pediatrics 91:160.

Lancet. 1992. Noticeboard. Vaccines quality control deficient. Lancet 340:1282.

Lasagna L. 1992. Introductory remarks. Cost containment and pharmaceuticals: Issues for future research. PharmoEconomics 1(Suppl.):1–76.

MedImmune, Inc. 1991. Annual Report. Gaithersburg, Maryland.

Merck & Co., Inc. 1991a. Annual Report. Rahway, New Jersey.

Merck & Co., Inc. 1991b. Form 10-K. Washington, D.C: Securities and Exchange Commission.

Mérieux A. 1992. Industrial Continuity and Response to Global Needs: A Challenging Paradox. Keynote address. Second Meeting of the Consultative Group of the Children's Vaccine Initiative, November 16-17, World Health Organization, Geneva.

National Research Council. 1992. U.S.-Japan Technology Linkages in Biotechnology: Challenges for the 1990s. Washington, D.C.: National Academy Press.

National Vaccine Injury Compensation Trust Fund. 1992. Materials provided at the Meeting of the Advisory Commission on Childhood Vaccines, Health Resources and Services Administration, Rockville, Maryland, December 2–3.

Office of Technology Assessment. 1991. Biotechnology in a Global Economy. Washington, D.C.

Oryx Press. 1992. Bioscan. Vol 6(Suppl. 4):1583. December. Phoenix, Arizona.

Pan American Health Organization. 1992. Progress in the worldwide polio eradication effort. EPI Newsletter 14(6):1.

Peter G. 1992. Childhood Immunizations. New England Journal of Medicine 327:1794–1800.

Pharmaceutical Manufacturers Association. 1990. Biotechnology Medicines. Washington, D.C.

Pharmaceutical Manufacturers Association. 1990. New Medicines in Development for Children. Washington, D.C.

Robbins A, Freeman P. 1988. Obstacles to developing vaccines for the Third World. Scientific American. November. pp. 126–133.

Saldarini RJ. 1992. Testimony before Senate Subcommittee on Appropriations. Childhood vaccine research and development issues. April 8. Washington, D.C.

Saldarini RJ. 1993. Testimony before the Subcommittee on Access to Immunization Services, National Vaccine Advisory Committee. A Public Hearing on the Economic and Commercial Underpinning of Vaccine Supply, February 24, Bethesda, Maryland.

Six H. 1992. Testimony before Senate Subcommittee on Appropriations. Childhood vaccine research and development issues. April 8. Washington, D.C.

SmithKline Beecham. 1991. Annual Report. Philadelphia.

Steele I. 1992. Vaccine price rise jeopardizes UCI. First Call for Children. A UNICEF Quarterly no.4:1–2.

Sugawara S. 1992. Biotech firms forming more strategic links: Young industry seeks support from mature corporations. October 19. Washington Post, Washington Business: p. 1.

Technology Management Group. 1993. Human Vaccine III. New Haven, Connecticut.

UNICEF. 1991a. Executive Board Action Item: Establishment of a Vaccine Independence Initiative. March 12. New York, New York.

UNICEF. 1991b. Executive Board: Universal Childhood Immunization, 1990, Progress Report. March 20. New York, New York.

UNICEF. 1992a. Vaccine Independence Initiative. Project Proposal for Funding by Interested Donors. July 13. New York, New York.

UNICEF. 1992b. Data regarding volume and price of purchased vaccines. Vaccine Supply Division. New York, New York.

U.S. Congress, House. 1986. Childhood Immunizations. A Report prepared by the Subcommittee on Health and the Environment, Committee on Energy and Commerce. September. Washington, D.C.

U.S. Congress, Senate. 1982. Hearing to Review Federal and State Expenditures for the Purchase of Children's Vaccines. Subcommittee on Investigations and General Oversight, Committee on Labor and Human Resources, July 22, Washington, D.C.

U.S. Department of Health and Human Services. 1991. Establishments and Products Licensed under Section 351 of the Public Health Service Act. March 1. Rockville, Maryland: U.S. Food and Drug Administration.

Vandersmissen W. 1992. Availability of quality vaccines: The industrial point of view. Vaccine 10:955–957.

Williams D. 1993. Testimony before the Subcommittee on Access to Immunization Services, National Vaccine Advisory Committee. A Public Hearing on the Economic and Commercial Underpinning of Vaccine Supply, February 24, Bethesda, Maryland.

World Almanac and Book of Facts. 1992. New York, New York: Pharos Books.

World Bank. 1993. World Development Report: Investing in Health. Washington, D.C.

World Health Organization. 1992. EPI for the 1990s. Geneva.

World Health Organization/Children's Vaccine Initiative. 1992a. CVI Forum. October. Geneva.

World Health Organization/Children's Vaccine Initiative. 1992b. Report of Second Meeting of the Consultative Group. November 16–17. Geneva.

World Health Organization/Children's Vaccine Initiative. 1992c. Task Force on Situation Analysis. November 16–17. Geneva.

Zoon KC Beatrice MG. 1993. New directions for FDA's Center for Biologics Evaluation and Research (CBER). New Drug Approvals in 1992. February. Washington, D.C.: Pharmaceutical Manufacturers Association.

5

Investing in New and Improved Vaccines

Vaccine development and manufacturing is an almost entirely commercial enterprise in the United States. Twenty years ago there were a dozen entities that made vaccines for U.S. children. Today, for a variety of reasons, nearly all the childhood vaccine used in this country are manufactured by four private companies (see Appendix H). At the beginning of 1993, there was only one supplier of oral polio vaccine (Lederle-Praxis Biologicals), one supplier of a combination measles-mumps-rubella vaccine (Merck and Co., Inc.), two companies that made a combination diphtheria and tetanus toxoids and pertussis vaccine (Connaught Laboratories, Inc., and Lederle-Praxis Biologicals) in the United States. The states of Massachusetts and Michigan manufacture combination diphtheria and tetanus toxoids and pertussis vaccines for their respective populations, but procure the oral polio vaccine from Lederle-Praxis Biologicals and the combination measles-mumps-rubella vaccine from Merck and Co., Inc.

The majority of basic research in the United States that leads to the development of new or improved vaccines is funded or conducted by the federal government, although a significant amount of research is conducted and funded by the private sector (Chapter 3). Product-oriented research and development (R&D) is conducted largely by biotechnology firms and established pharmaceutical companies. Although pharmaceutical companies have shown an interest in developing new and improved vaccines for domestic use, little effort has been expended to improving existing vaccines for use in the developing world (see Tables 4-11 and 4-12).

Established pharmaceutical firms currently devote approximately 5 percent of their total R&D expenditures to applied vaccine-related R&D, often building upon basic discoveries made through federally funded research (see Table 4-10). Over the last 10 years, biotechnology firms have emerged as a new force in the area of applied vaccine research and early-stage product development. However, as noted in Chapter 3, neither biotechnology firms nor the federal agencies involved in vaccine research currently have the capability of manufacturing vaccines on a large scale. This is also true for Massachusetts and Michigan, the only two states currently producing vaccines. Consequently, large-scale manufacturing capacity rests entirely with the large commercial manufacturers.

Generally, a commercial manufacturer begins the process of vaccine development when scientific research has yielded promising results and when "proof of principle" (the point in R&D when the feasibility of a particular product or process is determined) has been established. The decision to invest in this process takes into account two critical factors: the technical feasibility and complexity of developing the vaccine and market considerations. These market considerations include the likelihood of and anticipated rate of return on investment, the availability of patent protection (and freedom from third-party patent rights), and the potential costs of liability exposure.

Corporate R&D investment in human vaccines is often viewed less favorably than investment in drug-related R&D (DeBrock, 1983; Freeman and Robbins, 1991; Institute of Medicine, 1985; Pettinga, 1983). Unlike drugs, which may be used many times by the same patient over the course of several years, vaccines are designed to give long-lasting immunity after one or at most a few administrations. Although the benefit of vaccination to the individual is clear, there is a larger benefit of vaccination that accrues to society at large if a significant proportion of the population is immunized and herd immunity is achieved (see Chapter 2).

Compared with drugs, vaccines are disproportionately complex, both in terms of the technologies used to produce them and the skills needed to manage those technologies (Institute of Medicine, 1992). The analogy has been made that pharmaceutical manufacturing is similar to chemistry, whereas vaccine production is more like agriculture: drugs can be synthesized and put in tablet form within days to weeks; however, it can take a year or more, with complicated intervening steps, between the first culture of a vaccine product and its eventual use in a child.

Vaccine manufacturing also requires substantially greater investment in sophisticated and elaborate production facilities than is typically true for pharmaceutical production (Institute of Medicine, 1992). Vaccine manufacturing facilities must be upgraded on a regular basis, and the technicians and researchers who operate them must be particularly well trained and motivated to ensure that the production of vaccines meets or exceeds good manufacturing practice standards. Ongoing quality control is critical in vaccine manufacture, since tests of the final product may not detect certain deficiencies.

Even if the technological feasibility of a vaccine product is established, commercial manufacturers may be unwilling to pursue development. The anticipated costs associated with R&D may be too high, patent issues may be too complex, the licensing process may present unacceptable obstacles, and the risks of liability may appear too great.

MARKET CONSIDERATIONS

Private-sector vaccine manufacturers in the United States pursue the development of vaccines that are both technologically feasible and that have a profitable market in industrialized countries (see Table 4-12). No additional incentives are needed, provided that companies are assured an adequate return on their investments.

In some instances, a company may be willing to undertake the development of a vaccine that is needed primarily in the developing world, provided that there are predictable markets of sufficient size and profitability. Such markets include U.S. armed forces, U.S. travelers, and wealthy segments of indigenous populations. In other instances, the development of new vaccines or improvements in existing vaccines cannot be justified economically or legally by commercial vaccine manufacturers.

Commercial enterprises cannot be expected to engage fully in a venture, such as the Children's Vaccine Initiative (CVI), that does not offer much hope of a return on investment. The primary objective of any business corporation, including pharmaceutical companies, is to enhance returns for its shareholders (American Law Institute, 1992). The legal system once forbade corporations from diverting resources away from maximizing returns for any reason at all. For example, in 1919, the Michigan Supreme Court rejected an effort by Henry Ford to reduce the price of his cars to benefit consumers, articulating the then prevailing view on corporate responsibility: "A business corporation is organized and carried on primarily for the profit of the stockholders. The powers of the directors is to be exercised in the choice of means to attain that end, and does not extend to a change in the end itself, to the reduction of profits, or to the nondistribution of profits among stockholders in order to devote them to other purposes" (*Dodge v. Ford Motor Co.*, 204 Mich. 459, 507, 170 N.W. 668, 684, 1919). The legal system has evolved to accept that corporations "may devote a reasonable amount of resources to public welfare, humanitarian, educational, and philanthropic purposes" (American Law Institute, 1992). Many pharmaceutical firms donate pharmaceutical and biological products for medical and emergency needs and have, in many cases, made a major contribution to the enhancement of public health in the world. For example, Wyeth Laboratories (United States) contributed substantially to the eradication of smallpox through the donation of the bifurcated needle and Merck and Company, Inc., currently donates Ivermectin™ to a number of developing countries to treat onchocerciasis (river blindness). Corporate decisions that are consistent with laudable public policy objectives are often inconsistent with the interests of the shareholders, however. Corporations are not only constrained by law but also must withstand the scrutiny of their shareholders who, if they are unhappy with management's decisions regarding the use of corporate resources, may sell their stock (thereby driving the stock price down) or may seek to replace management altogether.

Without an expectation of adequate returns, it is unrealistic to expect commercial vaccine manufacturers to divert their resources in favor of what U.S. and international public health experts and world leaders may perceive to be a greater public good. As a result, commercial vaccine manufacturers cannot bear the sole responsibility for the development of high-risk, low-priced products such as those envisioned by the CVI.

Market Size

The pediatric vaccine market in the United States is as predictable as it is limited. The size of the market is defined by the birth cohort in the United States, roughly 4 million live births annually, and the number of visits children make to clinics or pediatricians to receive necessary booster shots.

There are two major classes of buyers of childhood vaccines: the public sector (including federal and state governments) and the network of private-sector physicians, hospitals, pharmacies, and clinics across the country. Over the last decade, the public sector has purchased an increasing share of the vaccines sold in the United States. Currently, a little more than half of all vaccines purchased in this country are bought with federal or state funds at federally negotiated prices (see Table 4-5). The current trend toward public-sector procurement of vaccines is of considerable concern to the large commercial manufacturers, particularly given calls for universal purchase of vaccines by the federal government (American Academy of Pediatrics, 1993; Liu, 1993; Marks, 1993; National Vaccine Advisory Committee; 1991) and the introduction of the Comprehensive Childhood Immunization Act of 1993 (H.R. 1640 and S. 732/733).

Industry representatives have indicated that they would find it difficult to maintain current investments in vaccine-related R&D if all childhood vaccines were purchased by the federal government (Douglas, 1992, 1993; Saldarini, 1992, 1993; Williams, 1993). They argue that the combined forces of a single government buyer and the unpredictability of the federal appropriations process would not provide companies with the confidence of a long-term, stable, and reliable infusion of the funds required to invest in highly innovative and risky vaccine R&D projects (Douglas, 1993). Furthermore, the vaccine manufacturers and some public health experts argue that a universal vaccine purchase policy would drive prospective companies out of the business altogether (Katz, 1993a,b; Williams, 1993). Others, however, believe that the effects of any large-scale federal procurement policy on the U.S. vaccine industry are not so clear (Edelman, 1993; Shalala, 1993). They assert that policies regarding pricing, funding for product development, and competitive production of vaccines could actually entice additional entries of companies into the U.S. vaccine industry (Edelman, 1993; Shalala, 1993).

Until quite recently, U.S. manufacturers have concentrated their sales efforts domestically. Merck & Co., Inc., and Lederle-Praxis Biologicals have now initiated efforts to market their vaccines in Europe and, more recently, the Confederation of Independent States. Merck has also bid on international tenders for hepatitis B vaccine sales in a number of foreign countries and is setting up a facility to produce hepatitis B vaccine in the People's Republic of China.

Despite some level of interest in certain overseas markets, U.S. vaccine manufacturers have expressed little interest in becoming involved in the high-volume, low-price market offered by the United Nations Children's Fund (UNICEF) and the Pan American Health Organization (PAHO) (Institute of Medicine, 1986, 1992). It has been suggested that the reason that U.S. companies do not bid for UNICEF and PAHO contracts is that it is illegal for U.S. commercial manufacturers to sell vaccines at prices lower than those that they charge the U.S. government (Institute of Medicine, 1992). However, government procurement regulations do not stipulate that the U.S. government receive the "best price." It would appear that much of the reluctance stems from the negative publicity that accompanied revelations some 10 years ago that U.S. vaccine makers were supplying vaccines to PAHO and individual developing countries at prices significantly lower than those charged the U.S. government. Speaking to a representative of a major vaccine manufacturer at a congressional hearing, Senator Paula Hawkins argued, "How can you justify charging nearly three times as much to the U.S. government as you did to foreign countries, and then the next year again submitting a bid also substantially below Federal U.S. prices?" (U.S. Congress, Senate, 1982). Indeed, the last time that a U.S. vaccine manufacturer bid on a UNICEF tender was in 1982, following the aforementioned congressional hearing.

Even though U.S. vaccine manufacturers do not supply vaccines to UNICEF or PAHO for distribution to the developing world, U.S. companies continue to be accused of marketing vaccines overseas at prices well below those they charge to the U.S. government. Indeed, in announcing his new childhood immunization initiative on February 12, 1993, President Clinton said, "I cannot believe that anyone seriously believes that America should manufacture vaccines for the world, sell them cheaper in foreign countries, and immunize fewer kids as a percentage of the population than any nation in this hemisphere but Bolivia and Haiti" (Clinton, 1993).

Intellectual Property

For the purposes of this report, intellectual property rights include patents, patent applications, and know-how. Know-how involves confidential information (e.g., trade secrets) and can be embodied in tangible items like tissue cultures and their genetic components as well as in less tangible forms, such as an oral disclosure of information. (see Appendix A). In vaccine development and manufacture, know-how is as important as patent considerations.

Patent Rights and Limitations

Pharmaceutical and biotechnology companies rely on patents to exclude others from unfairly reaping the rewards of their investments in research and to protect the markets they serve.

The protection granted under patent laws is a 17-year "right to exclude others from making, using, or selling the invention throughout the United States" (35 USC § 154 (Supp. 1982)). In return for that right, the patentee is required to disclose, in detail, the subject matter of the invention. The owner of a patent is not granted the right to exclude others from using the information disclosed in the patent application to produce and patent a noninfringing, new, different, and better product or process. Therefore, disclosure not only promotes additional R&D but also discourages unnecessary duplication of research.

The patent owner is granted a 17-year right to exclude others from making, using, or selling the patented invention in the United States. The patent right does not extend beyond the United States, and if protection is desired in foreign countries, patents must be applied for there as well. The patent owner receives no affirmative right to make, use, or sell the claimed invention. In fact, a patent owner may find that practicing the invention infringes upon another party's previously issued patent. In this case, a patent owner must be authorized by the holder of the previously issued patent to use the owner's invention. For example, if a patentable improvement were made on a patented vaccine, the inventor of the improvement would need permission from the first-generation patent holder of the vaccine to make, use, or sell the improved vaccine.

There is no requirement that one use or license a patented invention, nor would one lose a U.S. patent for failing to use it. One can own a patent, never use it, and still exclude everyone else from making, using, or selling it. In contrast, most other countries impose a requirement that a patent owner must use or license a patented invention within a defined period of time.

A patent license is a transaction in which the patent owner gives permission to another party to use his or her patent. Patent licenses can be sought prospectively, before investment in product development, or after the product is in hand and on the market. Taking the former approach may require more licenses to cover applications that might become patented, as well as those that are already patented. Awaiting product completion may give the patent holder greater leverage, in view of the developer having extended itself, and the developer could run the risk of losing all by injunction unless a steep price is paid.

Patents and Vaccines

Historically, vaccines have been perceived to be more difficult to patent than drugs. This perception is changing in the wake of advances in biotechnology and the spur of *Diamond v. Chakrabarty*, 447 U.S. 303,309 (1980), a landmark legal decision that affirmed the patentability of microbial life forms and "anything under the sun that is made by the hand of man." Increasingly, layers of patent applications are filed—often by different groups and companies—on techniques, components, and genetic subassemblies of microbial systems used in the manufacture of biologics. The explosive growth of biotechnology and in the number of companies engaged in it has led to a mushrooming of patent applications and patents.

Under U.S. law, pending patent applications are held in confidence until they are granted (see Appendix A). By comparison, if corresponding applications are lodged overseas, they are typically "laid open" to public examination 18 months after the first filing. Even in this event, it is not possible to track the progress of corresponding U.S. applications through proceedings in the U.S. Patent and Trademark Office, or even to learn whether they have been abandoned.

The net effect of these patent-related concerns is to increase the level of uncertainty, and risk, surrounding investments in vaccine-related R&D. The list of potential unknowns is daunting and includes the type of patent protection a company or its competitor might win, how courts will decide competing claims, the number of third-party patents that might ultimately overlay a particular product, and whether necessary licenses can be assembled at a reasonable cost. Thus, when the possibility of financial reward is perceived to be low, as might be true for CVI vaccines, risk aversion runs high.

Infringement

An individual or company who violates the patent owner's rights is liable for patent infringement. If patent rights have indeed been violated, the owner is entitled to an injunction—a court order that prohibits an infringer from continuing to make, use, or sell the invention. The issuance of injunctive relief is within the discretion of the court. The Patent Act also authorizes an award of "damages adequate to compensate for the infringement, but in no event less than a reasonable royalty for the use made of the invention by the infringer" (35 USC § 284). The court may increase the damages awarded by as much as threefold and may award interest and costs. This is usually done when the infringement was willful.

As noted above, prospective infringement of valid patents can be prevented by injunctions, but the courts may withhold an injunction when not doing so would be contrary to public health or needs. Requests for injunctions are sometimes refused when the patent infringer is meeting a public health need that would otherwise go unserved. To grant such an injunction in private litigation is entirely within the discretion of courts, however, and few private companies are willing to bank on the court's unwillingness to grant such a remedy. No injunctive relief is possible when the invention is used "by or for the United States" (28 USC §1498). This exception to injunctive relief is broad. As the Patent Act states: "For the purposes of this Section, the use or manufacture of an invention described in and covered by a patent of the United States by a contractor, a subcontractor, or any person, firm, or corporation for the Government and with the authorization or consent of the Government, shall be construed as use or manufacture for the United States" (28 USC §1498). Here, the patentee's only remedy is an action against the government in the U.S. Claims Court for "reasonable and entire compensation" (28 USC §1498).

LIABILITY

There is always the risk that a drug or vaccine will cause unwanted and potentially serious health effects. All pharmaceutical companies market products with the knowledge that they may be sued for an adverse reaction months to years after the product is used. Most firms accept this risk and adjust the prices of their products upward to cover their perceived liability exposure (Institute of Medicine, 1985).

In the case of vaccines, a manufacturer's evaluation of liability risks depends in part on whether the vaccine would be used only in developing countries or whether it would be marketed in the United States, a notoriously litigious society. In general, liability concerns appear to be of less concern in developing-country markets. Foreign plaintiffs do sometimes sue U.S. pharmaceutical manufacturers in U.S. courts for injuries allegedly caused by products sold abroad, however. The determination as to whether such claims can be maintained in the U.S. courts is made on a case-by-case basis.

Compared with other pharmaceuticals, vaccines are unique in ways that may cause manufacturers to assess their risks and benefits differently. For example, vaccines are administered to healthy people, and as a result, adverse reactions are far more noticeable and less tolerated by the vaccinee and family. In addition, when the injured person is a child with many potential years of life left, settlements from litigation over injury resulting from receipt of a childhood vaccine can be much larger than those from other products that are used primarily by adults (Institute of Medicine, 1985; Wendy K. Mariner, Boston University School of Public Health, personal communication, 1992;).

Liability exposure was cited by many vaccine makers as the primary reason they exited the vaccine business in the 1970s and early 1980s (U.S. Congress, House, 1986). There is some reason to believe that the generally lower rate of return for most vaccines produced during that period, as well as the U.S. Food and Drug Administration's stringent requirements for demonstration of vaccine efficacy, also influenced companies' decisions to withdraw from the market.

The National Vaccine Injury Compensation Program (NVICP), authorized by the U.S. Congress in 1986 and implemented in 1988, was an attempt both to compensate the families of children adversely affected by government-mandated vaccines and to shore up the vaccine industry by eliminating liability risk through the imposition of a vaccine excise tax (Public Health Service Act, 1987; 100 Stat. 3756, codified as Title XXI of the Public Health Service Act at 42 USC 300aa-1 et *seq.* (Supp. V 1987); the Compensation Program is codified as Subtitle 2 of Title XXI, 42 USC 300aa-34). The excise tax was removed by the Secretary of the Treasury on

January 1, 1993, when a bill unrelated to the NVICP but containing language that would have extended the tax was vetoed by President Bush. The trust fund into which the excise taxes were paid had a balance of about $620 million at the beginning of 1993.

It is too early to assess the program's impact on future cases of liability against individual manufacturers, and it is not entirely clear that the compensation program is having the desired impact on the number of vaccine manufacturers in the business (see Appendix B). Despite the apparent drop in vaccine-related lawsuits and despite the increased activity in vaccine-related R&D (see Chapter 4), none of the companies that dropped out of vaccine manufacturing in the United States in the 1970s and 1980s have returned. However, as noted in Chapter 4, foreign companies, many of whom have traditionally shied away from the U.S. vaccine market, appear to be readying themselves to enter the U.S. market, either by applying for FDA licenses for their products or by entering into alliances with other companies and entities that currently hold U.S. product licenses.

REFERENCES

American Academy of Pediatrics. 1993. Childhood Vaccine Act. January. Washington, D.C.

American Law Institute. 1992. Principles of Corporate Governance. March 31. Philadelphia.

Clinton WJ. 1993. Statement at the Fenwick Center Health Clinic, Arlington, Virginia. February 12.

DeBrock L. 1983. The Domestic Vaccine Industry: The Economic Framework. Paper presented at the Institute of Medicine Conference on Barriers to Vaccine Innovation, November 28–29. Washington, D.C.

Douglas GR. 1992. Testimony before the Senate Subcommittee on Appropriations. Childhood vaccine research and development issues. April 8. Washington, D.C.

Douglas GR. 1993. Testimony before the Senate Labor and Human Resources Committee and the House Subcommittee on Health and the Environment. April 21. Washington, D.C.

Freeman P, Robbins A. 1991. The elusive promise of vaccines. The American Prospect. Winter:80–90.

Institute of Medicine. 1985. Vaccine Supply and Innovation. Washington, D.C.: National Academy Press.

Institute of Medicine. 1986. Proceedings of a Workshop on Vaccine Supply and Innovation. Report for the Subcommittee on Oversight and Investigations of the Committee on Energy and Commerce. U.S. House. August. Washington, D.C.

Institute of Medicine. 1992. Proceedings of Working Groups on The Children's Vaccine Initiative: Planning Alternative Strategies Towards Full U.S. Participation. June. Washington, D.C.

Katz S. 1993a. Could the childhood vaccine act be bad? Letter to the Editor. Pediatrics 91:160.

Katz S. 1993b. Testimony before the Subcommittee on Access to Immunization Services, National Vaccine Advisory Committee. A Public Hearing on the Economic and Commercial Underpinning of Vaccine Supply, February 24, Bethesda, Maryland.

Koop CE. 1993. In the dark about shots. February 10. Washington Post, p. A21.

Liu J. 1993. Testimony before the Subcommittee on Access to Immunization Services, National Vaccine Advisory Committee. A Public Hearing on the Economic and Commercial Underpinning of Vaccine Supply, February 24, Bethesda, Maryland.

Marks P. 1993. Vaccines available but many children go without. February 14. New York Times, Metro Section, p. 1.

Mazzuca L. 1992. Shot through with problems. August 24. Business Insurance, p. 1.

National Vaccine Advisory Committee. 1991. The Measles Epidemic: The Problems, Barriers, and Recommendations. Journal of the American Medical Association. 266(11):1547–1552.

Pettinga CW. 1983. Vaccine innovation and the private sector. Paper presented at the Institute of Medicine Conference on Barriers to Vaccine Innovation, November 28–29. Washington, D.C.

Saldarini RJ. 1992. Testimony before the Senate Subcommittee on Appropriations. Childhood vaccine research and development issues. April 8. Washington, D.C.

Saldarini RJ. 1993. Testimony before the Senate Labor and Human Resources Committee and the House Subcommittee on Health and the Environment. April 21. Washington, D.C.

Shalala DE. 1993. Testimony before the Senate Labor and Human Resources Committee and the House Subcommittee on Health and the Environment. April 21. Washington, D.C.

U.S. Congress, House. 1986. Childhood Immunizations. A Report prepared by the Subcommittee on Health and the Environment, Committee on Energy and Commerce. September. Washington, D.C.

U.S. Congress, Senate. 1982. Hearing to Review Federal and State Expenditures for the Purchase of Children's Vaccines. Subcommittee on Investigations and General Oversight, Committee on Labor and Human Resources. July 22. Washington, D.C.

Williams DJ. 1993. Testimony before the Senate Labor and Human Resources Committee and the House Subcommittee on Health and the Environment. April 21. Washington, D.C.

6

Stages of Vaccine Development

For the purposes of this chapter, the process of vaccine research and development (R&D) is described as if the process occurs in an ordered, chronological fashion. In this somewhat simplified view, vaccine research begins only after a careful assessment of public health priorities. Work conducted in the basic research laboratory forms the scientific foundation for all subsequent investigation. Applied R&D then moves to the clinical research setting, and from there to pilot production and full-scale manufacture. The vaccine must then be purchased, distributed, and used. Finally, a surveillance system is established to monitor immunization coverage, efficacy, and any adverse health effects related to vaccine administration. The surveillance system also may detect fluctuations in disease incidence or new disease entities requiring a realignment of public health priorities.

In reality, the stages of vaccine development are not so neatly divided. For instance, although basic research is the starting point, it does not end when applied R&D begins; basic research findings continue to inform the process of vaccine development, even during clinical testing. Likewise, findings at the applied and clinical levels feed observations and questions back to the basic research laboratory.

In Chapter 5, the committee examined broad questions of market potential and technical feasibility, both of which influence the decision to invest in the development of new or improved vaccines. After this decision to invest in a vaccine is taken, vaccine manufacturers are then frequently faced with a range of impediments as a product moves through the successive steps of development.

This chapter describes the various phases of vaccine development and a number of obstacles that can arise in this process. These barriers can discourage initial investment or prevent the vaccine from advancing beyond a certain stage. At every step, commercial manufacturers weigh the likelihood of product success against its market potential.

PRIORITY SETTING

The decision-making process for the development and production of vaccines should be guided by an assessment of critical public health needs. Priorities should be established and the desired vaccine characteristics should be defined. In this way, the vast resources of the U.S. and international public and private sectors can be directed to a set of common and complementary goals.

There have been major efforts over the past decade to establish priorities for vaccine development (Institute of Medicine, 1986a,b; National Institute of Allergy and Infectious Diseases, 1992a,b; World Health Organization, 1991; World Health Organization/Children's Vaccine Initiative, 1992c). As discussed in Chapter 3, much of the basic vaccine research conducted by the National Institute of Allergy and Infectious Diseases (NIAID) targets the development of priority vaccine candidates identified in 1986 by the Institute of Medicine (Institute of Medicine, 1986a,b; National Institute of Allergy and Infectious Diseases, 1992a,b), and much progress has been made (National Institute of Allergy and Infectious Disease, 1992b).

At present, new efforts are under way to develop priorities for vaccine R&D. The Task Force on Priority Setting and Strategic Plans of the World Health Organization's (WHO's) Children's Vaccine Initiative (CVI) recently completed a major cost-effectiveness assessment of vaccine-development priorities, and the WHO/United Nations Development Program's (UNDP) Program for Vaccine Development maintains a list of priority areas for vaccine development. In addition, the World Bank, as part of the World Development Report of 1993, *Investing in Health* (World Bank, 1993), is using Disability Adjusted Life Years to estimate the burden of disease and priorities for intervention.

Whatever priorities are set by the public sector, the ultimate decision to develop and manufacture a vaccine for general use in the United States rests entirely with the commercial vaccine manufacturers (see Chapters 3, 4 and 5 and Appendix H). Commercial manufacturers vigorously pursue the development of those products with market potential (see Chapter 4). Vaccines used exclusively in the developing world hold little promise of significant returns on investment, and companies are reluctant to invest in developing such high-risk and commercially unattractive products (see Chapter 5).

The committee believes that priority setting and characterization of desired vaccine products is a critical stage of vaccine development, particularly for vaccines of low commercial interest but acute public health need. In this regard, the committee urges all groups involved in vaccine R&D for international public health applications to focus on a common and complementary set of vaccine priorities.

BASIC AND APPLIED RESEARCH

The fundamental scientific advances that make vaccine development possible arise from basic research. The full implications and ultimate applications of discoveries made in the basic research laboratory may be unanticipated, even by the investigators involved. Basic research relevant to vaccine development includes such things as the identification and isolation of the protective antigens of a specific pathogen, methods for DNA cloning, the creation of new vector systems, and the development and immunologic evaluation of new adjuvant systems.

Basic research is conducted primarily by federally funded academic and government scientists. Once a basic scientific finding is thought to have significant and practical applications, the research moves on to applied R&D (the exploratory development phase). Much applied research and almost all product-development activity are conducted by private industry. Both biotechnology firms and vaccine manufacturers invest in developing new technologies to deliver and enhance the quality and efficacy of vaccines. Unfortunately, some CVI-specific vaccine technologies (e.g., heat stabilization of viral vaccines) are unlikely to be pursued by U.S. firms, because such technologies would have little comparative advantage in the domestic market. The committee believes that additional incentives can be provided to university-based researchers, commercial vaccine manufacturers, and biotechnology companies to stimulate the development of such technologies and their subsequent handoff from basic research to the product-development stages. Possible incentives are discussed in Chapter 7.

CLINICAL EVALUATION

Good vaccines must meet basic criteria of safety, purity, potency, and efficacy. When a product has completed preclinical studies (usually involving animal models) and the sponsor is considering clinical trials in humans, an Investigational New Drug (IND) application is submitted to the U.S. Food and Drug Administration (FDA). The IND application contains information on the vaccine's safety, purity, potency, and efficacy (see Appendix C). These parameters are then evaluated in clinical trials, which are usually carried out in four phases (Table 6-1). Phase I trials are short-term studies involving a small number of subjects and are designed primarily to evaluate the safety of the candidate vaccine, its ability to induce an immune response (immunogenicity), the optimal dose range, and the preferred route of administration to achieve the most effective immune response. Studies are usually conducted in individuals at low risk of acquiring natural infection in order to avoid confusing results.

Following the successful completion of phase I trials, phase II trials are conducted; these may involve up to hundreds of subjects. Phase II trials are usually double-blind studies with a placebo-control group; phase II trials expand the evaluation of the safety and immunogenicity of the vaccine and may include the responses of individuals at risk of acquiring the infection. For a treatable pathogen, trials can be conducted in susceptible adults under controlled conditions to assess the ability of the vaccine to confer protection against experimental challenge. The results of these pilot studies can provide the information necessary to proceed with phase III studies.

Phase III trials are usually conducted in a double- or single-blind, placebo-controlled, randomized manner and in hundreds to thousands of individuals at risk for acquiring the infection or disease. Because of the lengthy observation period that may be required, the longer-term safety of the vaccine can also be assessed in a large number of subjects. Such trials are expensive, require a well-developed health infrastructure and large study groups (sometimes in non-U.S. populations), and, as with all stages of clinical investigation, demand experienced personnel and laboratory capacity for surveillance. Additional expenses are incurred if testing of live attenuated or live recombinant vaccines requires isolation facilities for phase I and II trials. Study design, data collection, and analysis are all of critical importance for ensuring the quality of trial results for licensing a candidate vaccine.

Phase IV trials may be conducted after a product is licensed, as part of postmarketing surveillance. They provide information about the safety and effectiveness of the vaccine in the general population, usually under normal (nonstudy) conditions.

Clinical trials are time-consuming (sometimes taking years), complex, and costly. Clinical trials for CVI vaccines, which are targeted for infants and young children, will be more challenging and time-consuming than those for vaccines designed for adults and older children. The safety and immunogenicity of many CVI vaccines will need to be demonstrated in trials

TABLE 6-1 Characteristics of Clinical Phases of Vaccine Research

Phase	No. of Subjects	Purpose	Characteristics of Study Population
I	5 to 50	Assess safety, immunogenicity, and optimize dose schedule	Conducted in individuals at low risk for infection May require placebo-controlled, double-blinded, and randomized study design
II	25 to 1,000	Expand safety, immunogenicity, and optimize dose schedule	May include at-risk population Usually double-blinded, placebo-controlled, and randomized
III	100 to 10,000	Assess safety	Conducted in population specifically at risk for the infection Usually placebo-controlled and randomized study design
IV	100,000 to millions	Assess safety and effectiveness under field conditions and detect rare adverse events	Postlicensure vaccinated population Observational study design Case-control methodology or population-based data often employed

SOURCE: Adapted from *The Jordan Report*, National Institute of Allergy and Infectious Diseases, 1992a.

successful can CVI vaccines be tested in young seronegative infants. Given in adult volunteers and then in older children. Only if those studies prove safety and ethical considerations, efficacy studies in infants may not permit challenge with the naturally virulent organism, but may require documentation of the prevention of natural infection compared with that in a placebo-controlled group. This progression of trials through younger age groups can be a lengthier process than that for strictly adult trials.

CVI vaccines will probably have to be tested in international field sites, since many of these vaccines are intended to prevent diseases from which children in the United States do not suffer. Ethical principles applicable to research with children would argue against subjecting healthy children to the risks of investigational vaccines that, even if proved effective, will be of no benefit to them or even to children in the same population. In addition, a CVI vaccine tested in healthy children in the industrialized. world may not perform adequately under certain conditions of sanitation, malnutrition, and concurrent infection that exist in the developing world. To the committee's knowledge, there are very few field sites equipped to evaluate vaccines definitively in infants. Such sites require an epidemiologically well-characterized population, adequate clinical and laboratory infrastructures, political commitment, local expertise, and on-going epidemiological field studies.

The United States, through various government agencies, including the U.S. Agency for International Development, the Centers for Disease Control and Prevention, the U.S. Department of Defense, and the National Institutes of Health, has considerable resources for conducting and evaluating clinical trials. The committee encourages these agencies to expand and make their international resources available to public- and private-sector entities interested in developing and testing CVI-related products. New sites capable of conducting vaccine trials in infants may have to be established, preferably in association with existing activities.

LICENSURE

Vaccine manufacturers apply to the FDA for a license to manufacture a vaccine by submitting a Product License Application (PLA). The PLA describes the firm's vaccine manufacturing process, quality control, and the results of clinical studies documenting the vaccine's safety and efficacy. Manufacturers also submit a second document, the Establishment License Application (ELA) or ELA amendment, describing the facilities, equipment, and personnel involved in the manufacturing process. Vaccine manufacturers also have to satisfy the FDA that they have followed establishment licensing standards and current Good Manufacturing Practices, an extensive body of regulations for manufacturing pharmaceuticals and biologics (the full range of the regulatory aspects of vaccine development are discussed in Appendix C).

The FDA's Center for Biologics Evaluation and Research (CBER) has come under criticism from the U.S. Congress and the pharmaceutical industry for the length of time–approximately 3 years–that it takes to approve PLAs and ELAs. Lengthy approval times are due in part to a rapidly increasing number of applications, many of which are for technologically new products, in the face of a level budget and staffing. The work overload has also made it difficult for CBER staff to devote time to their ongoing research projects and to keep abreast of technological developments. Although application approval times are likely to shorten over the coming years, the licensing of biologics will almost always be a lengthy process because of the high safety and efficacy standards that are required. Considerable time is required to acquire substantiating data from clinical trials, and this process is especially time-consuming for new vaccines.

In an effort to promote faster approval of drugs and vaccines, the Drug User Fee Act (P.L. 102-571) was passed in 1992. Under the new law, pharmaceutical companies must submit fees of $100,000 or more per application. The additional funds will be used to boost the size of FDA's application review staff from the current level of 1,000 to 1,600 over 5 years (Kessler, 1992). CBER's share of the increase will be on the order of 300 staff members. By 1997, the agency expects to review and act on completed PLAs and ELAs for priority applications within 6 months; for standard applications, the review time will be no more than 1 year (Kessler, 1992a). There is some concern that companies will be unwilling to pay the fees for CVI vaccines, which will be used primarily in the developing world. The user-fee law also may force the FDA to curtail many of its international activities and, instead, focus on domestic issues. FDA staff currently serve on international committees and work on bilateral projects to advise selected developing countries on regulatory policies. The committee addresses some of these regulatory concerns in Chapter 7.

PRODUCTION

Pilot Production

Pilot production, which occurs at or near the end of the applied research phase, is a critical stage in vaccine development. It is during the pilot manufacturing stage that vaccine is produced for use in safety and immunogenicity tests. Pilot vaccine manufacturing should be performed by using current Good Manufacturing Practices and, ideally, should be done on a scale sufficiently large to closely simulate the scale that will be used in commercial manufacturing. This is important if technical problems during scaleup are to be avoided, to ensure that the vaccine lots used in human efficacy studies will be similar to those produced commercially, and to facilitate the transfer of vaccine technology to commercial vaccine manufacturers in the United States and/or to manufacturers in developing countries.

As part of the IND application process, pilot lots of vaccine are produced (using Good Laboratory Practices or, preferably, current Good Manufacturing Practices). Careful attention is paid to controlling the steps of production so that a consistent product is obtained each time. Procedures for process control and for final product characterization are developed and then performed on each lot.

The United States has a limited number of facilities that are capable of producing pilot lots of vaccine and that meet Good Laboratory Practices and current Good Manufacturing Practices standards. In the public sector, only the Michigan and Massachusetts departments of public health, as well as the U.S. Department of Defense (through a contract with the Salk Institute in Swiftwater, Pennsylvania, and using a newly reconstructed plant at the Forest Glen section of the Walter Reed Army Medical Center have the capability of producing pilot lots of viral, bacterial, and antiparasitic vaccines (Table 6-2).

Commercial vaccine manufacturers in the United States and Europe have the greatest capability of producing pilot lots of vaccine, but their facilities are often oversubscribed and precedence is given to products with the highest commercial potential. Indeed, the private sector has shown little interest in producing pilot lots of developing-world vaccines for such organizations as the UNDP/World Bank/WHO Special Program for Research and Training in Tropical Diseases (United Nations Development Program/World Bank/World Health Organization Special Program fo Research and Training in Tropical Diseases, 1992). Vaccines that have an immediate and defined market and less risk of technical failure, such as influenza vaccines, will always command priority in the vaccine development and production pipeline of commercial vaccine manufacturers. Indeed, a recent U.S. Department of Defense phase II trial of a candidate malaria vaccine had to be scaled back to involve half the number of volunteers needed because the Department of Defense's commercial partner could not produce a second batch of vaccine because other vaccine candidates had priority for the company's pilot facilities (Jerald C. Sadoff, Walter Reed Army Institute of Research, personal communication, 1993). Indeed, for all practical purposes, commercial manufacturers' pilot production facilities

TABLE 6-2 Existing U.S. Public-Sector Vaccine Development and Manufacturing Facilities

Activities	DOD	MA	MI	NIH	Salk
Basic research	Yes	Yes	No	Yes	No
Production research and development					
Bacterial vaccines	Yes	Yes	Yes	Yes[a]	Yes
Viral vaccines	Yes	No	Yes	Yes[b]	Yes
Parasitic vaccines	Yes	No	No	Yes	Yes
Pilot vaccine manufacturing					
Bacterial vaccines	Yes	Yes	Yes	Yes	Yes
Viral vaccines	Yes	No	Yes[c]	Yes[b]	Yes
Parasitic vaccines	Yes	No	No	No	Yes
Quality control/quality assurance	Planned	Yes	Yes	No	Yes
Total annual budget	~$55m	~$8m	~10m	~960m[d]	~9.6m
Budget for vaccine research and development	~20m	~1.5m	~1.5m	~130m[d]	~1m
Capacity for large-scale manufacture	Yes	Yes	Yes	No	Some

NOTE: DOD, U.S. Department of Defense; MA, Massachusetts Department of Public Health Biologics Laboratories; MI, Michigan Department of Public Health Biologics Laboratories; NIAID, National Institute of Allergy and Infectious Diseases; Salk, Salk Institute (Swiftwater, Pennsylvania); m, million.

[a] National Institute of Child Health and Human Development.
[b] Contracts out.
[c] Rabies vaccine.
[d] Figure represents NIAID budget only.

have been unavailable to multilateral organizations and members of the public sector seeking to develop those vaccines that have a high technical risk and that are likely to be of limited commercial value (Tore Godal, Director, UNDP/World Bank/WHO Special Program for Research and Training in Tropical Diseases, personal communication, 1993).

Contracting out pilot production to specialized private-sector firms is a limited option for both private-sector firms and the public sector, including the U.S. Department of Defense. Only a handful of small privately held firms in the United States can make peptides according to current Good Manufacturing Practices, and even fewer have filling and bottling capabilities, with the consequence that filling and bottling must be completed elsewhere. Many private companies, most particularly start-up biotechnology companies, are reluctant to contract pilot production to others for fear of losing proprietary technology and know-how (Lance Gordon, President, ORAVAX, personal communication, 1993). The end result of the shortage of vaccine pilot production facilities is considerable delay (sometimes years) in producing pilot batches of required vaccines.

The difficulties and delays associated with contracting out pilot production and bottling and filling prompted the U.S. Department of Defense to reconstruct its own pilot production facility at Forest Glen, Maryland. Even though the Forest Glen facility is not yet operational, WHO, the U.S. Agency for International Development, several institutes at the National Institutes of Health, and several small biotechnology firms are entering into agreements with the Department of Defense to access the pilot production capability (Jerald C. Sadoff, Walter Reed Army Institute of Research, personal communication, 1993). Indeed, it appears that the Forest Glen facility will be oversubscribed before it becomes fully operational.

In the committee's view, the lack of pilot production facilities is a major bottleneck in the development of vaccines in general, and CVI vaccines in particular. This concern is addressed in the committee's recommendations in Chapter 7.

ScaleUp and Full-Scale Manufacture

Manufacturers confront one of the most difficult, complex, time-consuming, and resource-intensive aspects of vaccine development when the decision is made to take a vaccine produced in small amounts in a pilot facility and to scale up production to commercial levels.

In the bench-level laboratory, scientists can work readily with vaccine produced in 1- to 10-liter bioreactors. Transferring production to the pilot scale of 50- to 100-liter volumes, however, is not simply a matter of increasing the size of the reaction vessel. The behavior of the microorganisms, biochemical and physiological interactions, and the rate of yield are among a number of variables that must be validated at each point in the scaleup process to ensure that the product is equivalent to that developed on the small scale.

Manufacturing high-quality and consistently potent vaccines on a large scale (500 liters or more) is a challenging process, even for well-established pharmaceutical firms. For example, the recent scaleup of a *Haemophilus influenzae* type b conjugate vaccine (Hib-CV) and a Hib-CV–diphtheria and tetanus toxoids and pertussis vaccine (DTP) combination was more difficult than anticipated (Centers for Disease Control and Prevention, 1992; Siber, 1992). Several manufacturers of single-component Hib-CV noted reductions in the immunogenicities of their vaccines that appeared to coincide with the scaleup process itself (Siber, 1992). In these recent cases, sophisticated physical and biochemical characterizations of the vaccines and animal testing did not predict the reduced immunogenicity.

The FDA is acutely aware of the problems inherent in scaleup for large-scale vaccine manufacture and strongly encourages manufacturers to produce clinical material for phase III studies in a commercial production facility. Given the paucity of such facilities in the United States, however, this is not always possible. In many instances, manufacturers must, prior to obtaining licensure, document that the material made in the pilot facility is equivalent to that produced in a commercial facility. Often, a clinical study must be conducted to prove this equivalence to the satisfaction of the FDA.

The FDA has recognized for some time that biotechnology and other small biologics companies are at a disadvantage when they try to obtain license approval, since many lack the facilities to manufacture biologics in their entirety on a commercial scale. To address this problem, the agency recently issued guidelines for firms seeking FDA approval for biologics manufactured under cooperative agreements (see Appendix C).

Vaccine Production in Developing Countries

The production of children's vaccines in developing countries is widespread and is likely to increase. Indeed, there is an increasing desire on the part of many nations to be self-sufficient vaccine producers. More than 80 percent of the children in the world are born in a country that produces one or more vaccines used in the Expanded Program on Immunization (EPI) (Amie Batson and Peter Evans, Expanded Program on Immunization, World Health Organization, personal communication, 1992; World Health Organization/Children's Vaccine Initiative, 1992a). Most of the bacterial vaccines used in EPI are produced in developing countries (Agency for Cooperation in International Health, 1992; Peter Evans, Expanded Program on Immunization, World Health Organization, personal communication, 1992). Almost 60 percent of the DTP in the world is manufactured in the country that uses it.

In June 1992, the World Health Assembly passed a resolution requiring every vaccine-producing country to have a national control authority and to be certified to sell EPI vaccines. It is not known how many countries that produce vaccines actually have a national control authority or other entity responsible for the quality control of locally produced vaccines, however. WHO's Division of Biologics publishes a number of technical reports and guidelines to help manufacturers of biologics produce safe and effective vaccine products. Although many local producers have formally adopted WHO's requirements for vaccine production, as a matter of practice, production standards are often established by the producer. Several U.S. agencies have developed programs to help countries improve the quality of locally produced vaccines. For example, the FDA, with support from the U.S. Agency for International Development, is working with India, Egypt, Saudi Arabia, and some members of the Confederation of Independent States to enhance the regulatory oversight of biologics.

The international transfer of CVI-related technology raises complex issues. Concerns have been raised about the safety and efficacy of vaccines currently produced in some countries (Agency for Cooperation in International Health, 1991; Hlady et al., 1992; Lancet, 1992; World Health Organization/Children's Vaccine Initiative, 1992a). Many of the vaccines proposed for development under the CVI will require more complex production techniques and manufacturing facilities than now exist in many parts of the world. The successful manufacture of effective, safe versions of these vaccines by the current set of producers thus may not be feasible in the short run, and some newer vaccine production technologies may not be amenable for transfer to developing countries.

The committee recognizes that the U.S. public and private sectors can play a critical role in supporting quality assurance, Good Laboratory Practices, and current Good Manufacturing Practices in vaccine-producing countries overseas. Such support could include the training of developing-country nationals in U.S. federal and state laboratories and established U.S. vaccine-manufacturing companies, as well as providing consultant support to manufacturers in developing countries in their efforts to meet current Good Manufacturing Practices.

RECOMMENDATIONS FOR USE

As part of the licensure process, recommendations for vaccine use are made by the vaccine manufacturer with the approval of the FDA and appear as part of the package insert. The package insert describes, among other things, the target group and dosage regimen, outlines contraindications, and provides information on side effects.

Recommendations for general vaccine use in the U.S. public sector are made by the Advisory Committee on Immunization Practices (ACIP) of the

Centers for Disease Control and Prevention. Separate and sometimes slightly different recommendations are produced by the Committee on Infectious Diseases of the American Academy of Pediatrics (AAP; the so-called Red Book committee) for use in the private sector (see Appendix G). Recommendations for use in the international sphere are often determined by WHO in conjunction with national governments.

ACIP recommendations are made on the basis of all available data regarding the vaccines under consideration presented to the ACIP both verbally and in written form. There have been instances in which some parents and pediatricians would have favored the ACIP and AAP going beyond the manufacturer's recommendations for use. For example, the first vaccine against *Haemophilus influenzae* type b (HibTITER) to be licensed in the United States was approved in December 1988 for use in children 18 to 60 months of age. It was not approved for use in infants until October 1990, when additional clinical studies were completed. The same scenario is now being played out with the acellular pertussis vaccine, which currently is approved for use only as a fourth booster dose. Although some may argue that there is little need to delay the use of vaccines in infants when trials in slightly older children indicate that they are safe and effective, it is impossible to predict whether vaccines will be as safe and effective in different age groups, especially in immunologically naive infants.

Recommendations to include new vaccines in the immunization schedule in the United States are made only after a vaccine has been licensed by the FDA. This can and has posed problems for vaccine manufacturers in the past when new vaccines are not recommended for integration into existing immunization schedules. For example, a polysaccharide pneumococcal vaccine for adult use was marketed in 1978. However, the ACIP's 1978 recommendations were so lukewarm that they effectively discouraged greater coverage among the elderly populations (Centers for Disease Control, 1978; Sisk and Riegelman, 1986). Because manufacturers can never be certain whether a licensed vaccine will be included among recommended immunizations, there have been suggestions that the ACIP and AAP make recommendations for use while the vaccines are in clinical trials. This would effectively commit the federal government to large-scale purchases of vaccine relatively early in the clinical testing phase and might give vaccine manufacturers the confidence to proceed with development (Institute of Medicine, 1986c).

There are several problems with this approach, however. First, most manufacturers need to assess the potential market for a product well before it reaches the clinical trial stage. Second, there are problems in recommending a vaccine for use when data concerning the target group are not available. Third, it is not possible to predict the outcomes of clinical trials, particularly in specific target groups tested in the later stages of a trial. Finally, FDA licensure and recommendations concerning an incompletely tested product cannot be predicted, nor expected.

PROCUREMENT

Worldwide, the United Nations Children's Fund (UNICEF) and the Pan American Health Organization (PAHO) are the largest purchasers of vaccines for use in the developing world (see Chapter 4). More than two-thirds of the vaccines supplied to UNICEF and PAHO are produced by European manufacturers; none are made by U.S. manufacturers.

The federal government is the largest purchaser of childhood vaccines in the United States. The public sector, through the Centers for Disease Control and Prevention (CDC) and the states, procures more than half of the vaccines used in this country, and the Army buys all of the vaccines used by the U.S. military (see Chapter 3). The private sector, through hospitals, clinics, and pediatricians, procures vaccines directly from the manufacturers. CDC's fiscal year 1992 vaccine purchases amounted to $154 million; the Army buys between $10 million and $30 million worth of vaccines annually.

In early 1993, the Clinton administration proposed that the federal government assume a larger role in purchasing childhood vaccines (the Comprehensive Childhood Immunization Act of 1993 [H.R. 1640 and S. 732 and S. 733]) (Clinton, 1993; Marks, 1993; Washington Post, 1993).

Currently, the CDC negotiates a federal purchase price for priority vaccines with key manufacturers. These public-sector rates are substantially lower than those listed in the private sector (see Chapter 4). The CDC then makes grants to the states to purchase the vaccines, passing on the lower prices. The federal government negotiates procurement contracts anew every year. Some have argued that the 1-year contracts serve as a disincentive to vaccine innovation, since companies have no guarantee that the products they develop and manufacture will be purchased for any substantial length of time. Others argue that extending the procurement contract could effectively shut out other manufacturers and lead to their exit from the vaccine business. Consequently, there is some concern that if the U.S. government emerged to be the sole purchaser of all pediatric vaccines, the little competition that exists among vaccine manufacturers in the United States would diminish even further. In addition, industry representatives have indicated that companies may be reluctant to invest in costly R&D if the government were to be the sole buyer (see Chapter 5) (Douglas, 1993).

DISTRIBUTION AND DELIVERY

Organizing effective and efficient vaccine distribution and delivery systems and communicating the importance of routine immunization to parents and health professionals are critical to ensuring adequate immunization coverage in the United States and around the globe. In much of the developing world, vaccines are distributed by ministries of health through EPI and by various nongovernmental organizations. The EPI has established a target to immunize 90 percent of children under 1 year of age by the year 2000. Achieving this level of immunization is anticipated to be an enormous challenge and is expected to require improved information and epidemiological surveillance systems to identify pockets of unvaccinated children and regions of persistent disease transmission, enhanced social mobilization, and additional resources to strengthen vaccine delivery. In addition, the introduction of new vaccine products into EPI will require close coordination among the implementing agencies.

SURVEILLANCE

Surveillance is key to monitoring important characteristics in a population in which a vaccine is introduced. These aspects include (1) the immunization rates attained in the targeted group, (2) the efficacy of the vaccine in preventing the disease, (3) the frequency and attributes of vaccine-related adverse reactions, and (4) the recognition of new infectious disease problems that require public health attention. Likewise, surveillance will be a fundamental component in monitoring the efficacies of CVI vaccines and any adverse reactions and contributing to the establishment of new vaccine development priorities.

Immunization Status

From the standpoint of disease control, making vaccines available is only the first step in ensuring adequate levels of immunization. For example, to receive the full benefit of vaccines, children must be immunized at specific times throughout infancy and into early adolescence. In a perfect world, every parent would keep track (or be notified by a health-care worker) of his or her child's immunization status and would make sure that the child received the needed vaccinations on time. This frequently does not happen in practice, however; indeed, as outlined in Chapter 2, many children in the United States under age 2 are underimmunized.

Some experts have suggested that the United States establish a computerized national vaccine registry (Freeman et al., 1993; Johnson, 1991), which allows for more efficient follow-up and notification of children who need vaccination by requiring uniform reporting. A national vaccine registry is proposed in congressional legislation (S. 732). In addition, the CDC is currently developing state-based plans for tracking immunication coverage (Walter Orenstein, Division of Immunization, Centers for Disease Control and Prevention, personal communication, 1993). Computerized tracking systems are likely to require large investments in new equipment and training and considerable behavioral changes among private health-care providers and the public at large.

Monitoring Effectiveness of Vaccines

For reasons that are not fully understood, vaccines that are very effective in preventing disease among infants in the industrialized world appear to be less efficacious in infants in different epidemiological settings. For example, both live oral polio vaccine and measles vaccine, both of which are comparable to effective products licensed in the United States, have tended to be less effective when used in areas highly endemic for these diseases, particularly in the developing world (Halsey et al., 1983; Patriarca et al., 1991). Under conditions of poverty, inadequate housing and sanitation, malnutrition, and concurrent infection, vaccines may not be as effective. On the basis of these and other experiences, scientists and public health experts must anticipate potential differences in vaccine efficacy when these vaccines are introduced in developing-world conditions. Appropriate and close monitoring of clinical trials under field conditions will be critical to the development and introduction of CVI vaccines.

Adverse Reactions

There is always a risk that a vaccine will have unwanted and possibly serious side effects (see Chapter 5). In November 1990, the Vaccine Adverse Events Reporting System (VAERS), implemented jointly by CDC and FDA, became operational. VAERS receives reports and monitors vaccine safety by examining the frequency of reported adverse events. Operated by a private contractor, VAERS obtains reports of adverse events from many different parties, including manufacturers, health-care professionals, state health coordinators, patients, and parents. VAERS is currently the only comprehensive vaccine safety surveillance system in the

United States.

The importance of long-term monitoring of adverse vaccine reactions was highlighted in late 1991 and early 1992. During that period, it was determined in follow-up studies that children who received the high-titer Edmonston-Zagreb strain of measles vaccine in certain locations in Africa and Haiti that are highly endemic for measles experienced high mortality rates compared with the mortality rates in those who received the standard Schwarz strain 6 to 10 months after being vaccinated (Garenne et al., 1991). Furthermore, and for reasons that are unclear to the scientific community, the mortality rate appeared to be higher in girls than in boys (Garenne et al., 1991). Because of these findings, WHO suspended the use of the high-titer measles vaccine in October 1992 while the mechanism of this adverse effect is under study (Weiss, 1992).

Setting Priorities for Vaccine Use and New Vaccines

A good surveillance system can lead to a realignment of priorities for vaccine development. Surveillance is also the principal way that the frequency of established diseases is monitored and outbreaks of new diseases are detected (Institute of Medicine, 1992). A good surveillance program can identify clusters of disease, track the demographic and geographic trends of an outbreak, and permit health-care professionals to assess and evaluate priorities for vaccine development. Without the data obtained through surveillance, it is impossible to know where disease control efforts should be targeted or to evaluate the impact of ongoing intervention efforts. Inadequate disease surveillance leaves policymakers and public health professionals with no framework for generating and executing policies to prevent or contain the spread of infectious disease.

REFERENCES

Agency for Cooperation in International Health. 1991. Report of the International Meeting on Global Vaccine Supply, May 23–26, Kumamoto, Japan.

Agency for Cooperation in International Health. 1992. Report of the Second International Meeting on Global Vaccine Supply, August 3–5, Tokyo, Japan.

Centers for Disease Control. 1978. Pneumococcal polysaccaride vaccine. Morbidity and Mortality Weekly Report 27:253–131.

Centers for Disease Control and Prevention. 1992. Advisory Committee on Immunization Practices Update: Report of PedvaxHIB lots with questionable immunogenicity. Morbidity and Mortality Weekly Report 41:878–879.

Clinton WJ. 1993. Statement at the Fenwick Center Health Clinic, Arlington, Virginia. February 12.

Douglas G. 1993. Testimony before the Senate Labor and Human Resources Committee and the House Subcommittee on Health and the Environment. April 21. Washington, D.C.

Freeman P, Johnson K, Babcock J. 1993. A health challenge for the states: Achieving full benefit of childhood immunization. Occasional paper. February. The John W. McCormack Institute of Public Affairs, University of Massachusetts at Boston.

Garenne M, Leroy O, Beau J, Sene I. 1991. Child mortality after high-titre measles vaccines: Prospective study in Senegal. Lancet 338:903–907.

Halsey NA, Boulos R, Mode F, Andre J, Bowman L, Yaeger RG, Toureau S, Rhode I, Boulos C. 1983. Response to measles vaccine in Haitian infants 6-12 months old: influence of maternal antibodies, malnutrition and concurrent illnesses. New England Journal of Medicine 313:544-9.

Hlady GW, Bennett JV, Samadi AR, Begum J, Hafez A, Tarafdar AI, Boring JR. 1992. Neonatal tetanus in rural Bangladesh: Risk factors and toxoid efficacy. American Journal of Public Health 82:1365-1369.

Homma A. 1992. Technology Transfer. Paper presented to the WHO/CVI Task Force on Priority Setting and Strategic Plans. Children's Vaccine Initiative, World Health Organization, Geneva.

Homma A, Knouss RF. 1992. Transfer of vaccine technology to developing countries: The Latin American experience. Paper presented to the NIAID Conference on Vaccines and Public Health: Assessing Technologies and Policies for the Children's Vaccine Initiative, November 5-6. Bethesda, Maryland.

Institute of Medicine. 1986a. New Vaccine Development, Establishing Priorities. Volume I. Diseases of Importance in the United States. Washington, D.C.: National Academy Press.

Institute of Medicine. 1986b. New Vaccine Development, Establishing Priorities. Volume II. Diseases of Importance in the Developing World. Washington, D.C.: National Academy Press.

Institute of Medicine. 1986c. Proceedings of a Workshop on Vaccine Supply and Innovation. Report for the Subcommittee on Oversight and Investigations of the Committee on Energy and Commerce. U.S. Congress, House. August. Washington, D.C.

Institute of Medicine. 1992. Emerging Infections. Washington, D.C.: National Academy Press.

Johnson KA. 1991. A National immunization registry: A proposal. Paper presented at the National Immunization Conference. June. Washington, D.C.

Kessler DA. 1992a. Letter to Representatives J. Dingell and N. Lent, September 14. U.S. Food and Drug Administration, Rockville, Maryland.

Kessler DA. 1992b. Testimony before Senate Subcommittee on Labor, Health and Human Services Committee on Appropriations. Childhood vaccine research and development issues. April. Washington, D.C.

Koop CE. 1993. In the dark about shots. February 10. Washington Post, p. A21.

Lancet. 1992. Noticeboard. Vaccines quality control deficient. Lancet 340:1282.

Marks P. 1993. Vaccines available but many children go without. February 14. The New York Times, Metro Section, p. 1.

National Institute of Allergy and Infectious Diseases. 1992a. The Jordan Report. Bethesda, Maryland.

National Institute of Allergy and Infectious Diseases. 1992b. Report of the Task Force on Microbiology and Infectious Disease. April. Bethesda, Maryland.

North American Vaccine. 1991. Annual Report. Beltsville, Maryland.

Patriarca P, Wright PF, John TJ. 1991. Factors affecting the immunogenicity of oral poliovirus vaccine in developing countries: review. Reviews in Infectious Diseases 13:926-939.

Siber G. 1992. Hib-DTP vaccine. Paper presented to the CVI Task Force on Priority Setting and Strategic Plans. Children's Vaccine Initiative, Geneva.

Sisk J, Riegelman RA. 1986. Cost-effectiveness of vaccination against pneumococcal pneumonia: An update. Annals of Internal Medicine 104:79–86.

Washington Post. 1993. Immunity for children. February 4, p. A20.

Weiss R. 1992. Measles battle loses potent weapon. Science 258:546–547.

United Nations Development Program/World Bank/World Health Organization Special Program for Research and Training in Tropical Diseases (TDR). 1992. Prospective thematic review (PTR) on directions and organization of TDR's research and development related to anti-parasite vaccines. March 2–3. Geneva.

UNIVAX Biologics, Inc. 1992. Annual Report. Rockville, Maryland.

World Health Organization. 1992. EPI for the 1990s. Geneva.

World Health Organization. 1991. Programme for Vaccine Development: A WHO/UNDP Partnership. December. Geneva.

World Health Organization/Children's Vaccine Initiative. 1992a. CVI Forum. October. Geneva.

World Health Organization/Children's Vaccine Initiative. 1992b. Meeting of the Consultative Group. November 16–17. Geneva.

World Health Organization/Children's Vaccine Initiative. 1992c. Report of Task Force on Priority Setting and Strategic Plans. November 16–17. Geneva.

7

A Strategy to Enhance U.S. Participation in the Children's Vaccine Initiative

The Children's Vaccine Initiative (CVI) seeks to harness new scientific technologies to advance the immunization of children throughout the world. The ideal CVI vaccine will require fewer doses and will be given near birth, be heat stable, effective against diseases for which vaccines are currently unavailable, and be affordable. Achieving the challenging vision of the CVI requires international commitment to the development and production of a new generation of vaccines. It is not only the health of those in the developing world that is at stake; the growing problem of immunization in the United States, especially among economically disadvantaged children, is a major concern.

Since the World Summit for Children in New York City in September 1990, many different countries and organizations are currently evaluating what each is most able and willing to contribute toward achieving the vision of the CVI. This committee was asked how best to enhance both U.S. public- and private-sector participation in the global CVI, recognizing that U.S. resources and scientific capabilities are significant and extensive.

The committee spent a great deal of time considering ways to enhance U.S. public- and private-sector participation in the CVI and to ensure that CVI vaccines are developed, manufactured, and made available to national immunization programs in developing countries. The committee evaluated three major strategies for achieving full U.S. participation in the CVI (see Appendix D). After much deliberation, the committee rejected two of these strategies as less than optimal. The first would have provided supplemental

128

funds to existing federal agencies to support CVI-related vaccine research and development and would have made changes in the way that the U.S. government participates in the purchase and delivery of vaccines for developing countries; another would have given the U.S. government a primary role in *all* stages of vaccine development, including large-scale manufacture and distribution. Although each approach was thought to have some merits, the committee felt that neither would capitalize on the unique skills, expertise, and capabilities in the private sector (both biotechnology firms and commercial vaccine manufacturers). In the committee's view, the success of U.S. participation in the CVI will depend ultimately on effective cooperation and collaboration among government, universities, and most critically, the private sector. The committee's recommended strategy, which is presented below, combines the most desirable characteristics of the two strategies outlined above and includes new elements designed to achieve the vision of the CVI.

A NATIONAL VACCINE AUTHORITY

In the committee's view, the United States, through both the public and private sectors, has the potential to contribute most significantly to the achievement of the goals of the global CVI through the development and production of CVI vaccines (Chapters 3 and 4). However, it has become clear to the committee that the fragmented system of vaccine research, development, and manufacture in the United States, which produces high-quality vaccines for the domestic market, is not likely to produce the vast majority of CVI vaccines (Chapters 3, 4, and 5) (Institute of Medicine, 1992). This is primarily because most CVI vaccines targeted to developing countries lack the market potential of vaccines intended for industrialized-country markets (Chapters 4 and 5). In this regard, the committee concurs with the findings of the Institute of Medicine report, *Emerging Infections* (1992) that an integrated process is required to ensure that needed vaccines that lack well-paying markets are developed and manufactured. In addition and over the course of this study, the committee identified a number of specific impediments that hinder the ability of the U.S. public and private sectors to pursue the development of vaccines in general, and of CVI vaccines in particular (Chapter 6). In the committee's view, a major bottleneck in the development of low-profit vaccines, such as those envisioned by the CVI, is the lack of pilot production facilities that are capable of meeting the U.S. Food and Drug Administration's standards of current Good Manufacturing Practices (Chapter 6). At present, pilot manufacture of vaccine products of low commercial value is postponed for months or even years in commercial facilities, while the small number of public-sector facilities remain oversubscribed.

In the committee's judgment, the optimal way to maximize U.S. public- and private-sector participation in the global CVI and ensure that needed vaccines are developed and manufactured for developing countries is to empower an entity to organize and manage an integrated process of CVI vaccine development, manufacture, and procurement that capitalizes on the skills and expertise in both sectors. At this time, no federal entity, with the possible exception of the U.S. Department of Defense, has the capability of undertaking the breadth and range of activities required to ensure the integrated development, production, and procurement of CVI vaccines. In the committee's view, the development of new and improved CVI vaccines is unlikely to occur unless there is an entity that has the mandate to manage and oversee the process from beginning to end. Because the private sector alone cannot sustain the costs and risks associated with the development of most CVI vaccines, and because the successful development of vaccines requires an integrated process,

the committee recommends that an entity, tentatively called the National Vaccine Authority (NVA), be organized to advance the development, production, and procurement of new and improved vaccines of limited commercial potential but of global public health need.

Mission

As envisioned by the committee, the overall mission of the NVA would be to foster the development of new and improved vaccines of limited commercial potential but global public health need through the maximal use of U.S. public- and private-sector expertise and resources. It would do this both by reducing the risks and costs to industry associated with vaccine development and by offering a variety of incentives to companies willing to undertake CVI vaccine development. The NVA would achieve its goals through a dynamic partnership with the public and private sectors, in which each contributes what it is best able and most willing to provide. The new entity would take advantage of the traditions of discipline and attention to the bottom line that are common to private industry and the accountability to societal needs embodied in the public sector.

To accomplish its mission, the NVA would operate as a product development unit. In conjunction with the global CVI, it would be involved in setting the priorities for and generating the desired characteristics of candidate CVI vaccines. The NVA would issue requests for proposals to encourage private-sector firms to develop targeted CVI products, and it would have an in-house capability to conduct applied research and development and manufacture pilot lots of vaccine. In the committee's judgment, this would overcome one of the major bottlenecks to the development of new and improved vaccine products, as identified and discussed in Chapter 6.

The NVA could have a collection of incentives at its disposal to encourage private-sector enterprises (both large commercial companies and development-stage firms) to participate in its vaccine-related activities. These include:

- guaranteed procurement of vaccine,
- research and development (R&D) tax credits,
- investment-tax credits for firms that undertake CVI activities,
- Small Business Innovation Research program grants for CVI products,
- Cooperative Research and Development Agreements (CRADAs),
- access to an NVA pilot production facility,
- financial assistance with clinical trials, and
- assistance in assembling intellectual property rights.

In its dealings with private-sector partners, the new entity could, as appropriate, retain the right to transfer technology it owns to developing countries. In addition, all such collaborative agreements with private-sector partners could include a clause to ensure that whatever products are developed would be affordable to markets in developing countries. Ensuring that vaccine products are affordable could be accomplished through a variety of mechanisms including: use of technological design (whereby the NVA would propose the use of simple, low-cost technologies in vaccine construction) or a pricing clause. Alternatively, the NVA could purchase vaccine products at one price, and sell them at another (thereby subsidizing the prices paid by the United Nations Children's Fund (UNICEF) and the Pan American Health Organization (PAHO) and providing higher returns to private developers and manufacturers, where appropriate).

The NVA would accomplish as much as possible by contracting with the private sector. However, to accelerate the development of CVI vaccines, the NVA would have its own vaccine development program, which would be called on to undertake product-related R&D, as needed. The committee believes that having a public-sector vaccine development and pilot manufacture facility would overcome a major bottleneck in the development of low-profit vaccines, including many of those envisioned by the CVI. The NVA pilot facility would be made available to newly emerging biotechnology companies, multilateral agencies and organizations, and public- and private-sector vaccine manufacturers that agree to develop CVI products. The NVA would support six broad areas of vaccine product development:

- vaccines used primarily in developing countries (e.g., shigella, cholera, salmonella, malaria, and dengue);
- improvements in existing vaccines that would not lead to a high market return but that would make them easier to distribute and administer or allow them to achieve immunity earlier in high-risk populations (e.g., heat-stable polio, single-dose controlled-release tetanus toxoid and other childhood vaccines, and a more immunogenic measles vaccine);
- development of simple, low-cost vaccine manufacturing technologies that could be easily transferred to vaccine manufacturers in developing countries (e.g., heat stability);
- exploitation of vaccine technologies that are nonproprietary and therefore of little interest to commercial manufacturers who desire market exclusivity;
- adaptation and introduction of currently available vaccines (e.g., pneumococcal conjugates) and new vaccines, including combination vaccines, to the developing world; and
- vaccines for which there are small or limited markets or that are otherwise unprofitable.

Functions

As a product development organization, NVA would be involved in nearly all aspects of vaccine innovation and development, from identifying priorities to arranging procurement (see the box "Functions of a National Vaccine Authority"). The concept behind the NVA is similar to the U.S. Department of Defense's (DOD) approach to vaccine development for U.S. military personnel.[1]

Setting Priorities and Product Characterization

The first step in vaccine development is to set the priorities and describe the desired characteristics for a target vaccine. Currently in the United States, no agency, public health committee, or other group sets the priorities or generates the desired characteristics for vaccines, particularly those envisioned in the CVI. The NVA would, in conjunction with the EPI, global CVI, representatives of U.S. government agencies, private-sector

---

Functions of a National Vaccine Authority

- Define the need
- Assess the market
- Establish priorities for U.S. CVI vaccine development in conjunction with the global CVI
- Characterize desired vaccine products
- Assemble intellectual property rights
- Advance CVI product development through the private sector
- Conduct in-house vaccine-related R&D
- Assist companies in the production of pilot lots of vaccine
- Support clinical testing and field trials of candidate vaccines
- Transfer CVI-related vaccine technology to developing-country manufacturers
- Train U.S. and overseas nationals in the principles of vaccine development, pilot manufacture, and quality control
- Arrange and contribute to the procurement of NVA vaccines
- Evaluate and redefine needs
- Represent the United States in international CVI forums, such as the Consultative Group

---

firms, and public health experts, set priorities and describe the desired characteristics of the vaccines to be advanced by the NVA. Given the likelihood of limited resources and the need to accelerate the development of CVI products, NVA would probably focus its initial product development efforts on just a few CVI vaccines.

Basic Research

The NVA would not conduct basic research but would draw on research and technologies developed in academic institutions and at the National Institutes of Health (NIH). The NVA could also provide resources to these institutions for research related to CVI vaccines and could help bring international vaccine development needs to the attention of the domestic scientific community.

Applied Research and Exploratory Development

NVA would have a core of scientifically trained staff that would be able to conduct applied vaccine-related R&D to meet the needs of CVI. NVA scientists would be actively involved in testing new approaches to vaccine construction, determining the feasibility of new technologies, and taking candidate vaccine products to the point of proof of principle (the point in R&D when the feasibility of a particular product or process is determined and product development can begin). In addition, NVA would be able to enter into CRADAs with private firms, giving the NVA access to additional staff, funding, and proprietary technologies. The incentive for firms to enter into CRADAs with NVA would be the right to manufacture or market successful vaccines or employ proprietary technologies developed under license for profitable markets.

Intellectual Property Rights

A key feature of NVA would be its capability to assemble patent and know-how rights. Because the promotion of the goals of CVI is a legitimate governmental purpose, NVA, as a part of the federal government, could retain the rights to patents and other forms of protection for products or processes developed with federal money. This could occur even if that work was conducted on its behalf by private parties. (The NVA could also take advantage of technology embodied in patents that were not the result of federally funded research. If CVI research or the supply of CVI products is "by or for" the U.S. government, nongovernmental patent holders would not be able to stop those activities through a preliminary or permanent injunction. Contractors serving the government's purposes would be protected from patent infringement suits. The only remedy available to this category of patent holder would be reasonable compensation, presumably a reasonable royalty from the U.S. government. As discussed in Chapter 5, since the NVA would be serving a need left unfulfilled by these patent holders, it is unlikely that such actions would proliferate. In any case, the size of the awards should be small.) The NVA would also be able to file patent applications both in the United States and foreign countries for vaccine-related inventions of the government. The NVA would not, however, be able to transfer technology or to require the transfer of technology it does not own, unless such action were allowed under the terms of a contract with the developer or patentee.

Product Development

The NVA would be a goal-oriented entity, targeting the development of a variety of specific CVI vaccines. Each vaccine would require a customized product development strategy. It is likely that some vaccines will be developed exclusively through a contracting mechanism. Other vaccines may require parallel tracks of development in the private sector and at the NVA. A few may require substantially more involvement by the NVA. In all of its work, the NVA would draw on technology developed through collaborative agreements and advances made through its CRADAs, by NIH, DOD, and other relevant agencies. The NVA would ensure that all applied research is consistent with the needs established at the outset of the priority-setting process and specified by potential end users of the vaccine products.

To accelerate the process of vaccine development, all R&D on NVA vaccines would be done under conditions of Good Laboratory Practices so that the results could be used in support of Investigational New Drug Applications and future Product License Applications. Manufacture of pilot lots of vaccine would be performed under Good Laboratory Practices and, whenever possible, current Good Manufacturing Practices on a scale sufficiently large to simulate closely the future manufacturing scale. This is important to avoid technical problems during scaleup, to ensure that the vaccine lots used in the pivotal efficacy studies will be similar to scaled-up vaccine lots, and to facilitate the transfer of vaccine technology to commercial or public sector vaccine manufacturers in the United States or public sector manufacturers in developing countries, or both. In addition, the NVA would be open to training both U.S. and overseas nationals in the principles of product development and manufacture of pilot lots of vaccines, including quality control and quality assurance.

Clinical Evaluation

The U.S. government, through the U.S. Agency for International Development (AID), the Centers for Disease Control and Prevention (CDC), DOD, and NIH, has considerable expertise in and resources for conducting clinical trials. Indeed, one of the most important ways that the U.S. government can share risk with the private sector is to organize, conduct, and evaluate clinical and field studies of new vaccines, especially in developing countries. As noted in Chapter 6, CVI vaccines pose additional challenges for clinical trials in that CVI vaccines will need to be tested in infants at international field sites. The NVA could enter into agreements with different federal agencies and multilateral organizations to evaluate candidate vaccines. To accomplish this activity, NVA staff could work with private-sector companies to design phase I studies in the United States, although most such firms may want to design and carry out those studies themselves. It is more likely that NVA scientists, in conjunction with staff at other relevant agencies, will play a greater role in later-phase studies and in forming collaborative relationships with ministries of health in developing countries.

Regulation

The U.S. Food and Drug Administration (FDA) is the U.S. government entity charged with ensuring the safety and efficacy of vaccines. The NVA could enter into interagency agreements with the FDA to conduct R&D, develop new product standards, and assist in technology transfer. The NVA might also work with the FDA to develop quality control and quality assurance methods that could be adapted to conditions that exist in the developing world. Most private-sector collaborators will develop production methodologies in line with accepted quality control standards. The NVA, which would have some expertise in regulatory affairs, could serve as a link with the FDA and between vaccine development companies in the United States, foreign regulatory authorities involved in vaccine licensing, and international agencies such as the World Health Organization (WHO). In addition, the NVA could contribute to or the FDA could waive the user fees that would be borne by companies seeking to license CVI vaccines (see Chapter 6).

Manufacture

Optimally, vaccines developed by the NVA and its private-sector partners would be licensed to public or commercial manufacturers in the United States. In instances in which there is no U.S. interest in manufacturing a vaccine, the NVA could elect to transfer technology to a foreign public-sector manufacturer, provided that the country upholds patents. Vaccines developed by or with the support of the NVA could be sold to public health departments in the developing world, to international agencies, such as UNICEF, or to commercial distributors in the developed world.

Procurement

In the United States, public-sector vaccine purchases fall under the aegis of CDC and DOD. Internationally, UNICEF and PAHO negotiate and manage the procurement of large amounts of vaccine for use in the developing world. The NVA will need to work closely with the global CVI, developing countries, AID, UNICEF, PAHO, WHO, and others to ensure that the vaccines it develops will meet their needs. The NVA could agree to buy a predetermined volume of vaccine, on the basis of projected needs in the target population, at a predetermined price. Or, alternatively, the NVA could act as a broker to put together the necessary funding from a variety of sources. Such arrangements could initially run for 3 to 5 years, but they could be negotiated for a longer term.

The guaranteed vaccine procurement mechanism considered above closely resembles the DOD procurement process. During the 1950s and 1960s, DOD procurement played a critical role in launching a number of small start-up firms in the semiconductor and computer electronics industries (e.g., Texas Instruments and Fairchild Semiconductor, the forerunner of the Intel Corporation and many others). By providing large purchase orders to producers of semiconductors that met its specifications, the DOD enabled fledgling producers to expand their revenues relatively rapidly. These producers would have found it much more difficult to enter commercial markets for their devices, because these markets are associated with much higher marketing and distribution costs. Numerous analyses of the semiconductor and other high-technology industries have argued that the effects of DOD procurement were more important than the effects of DOD research and development contracts on the entry and growth of new firms in these markets (Flamm, 1987; Levin, 1982; Mowery et al, 1991).

To the extent that the risk and financial burden of vaccine development and clinical trials have been assumed by the public sector and the market size has been defined, it would become possible to negotiate licensing agreements that guarantee lower vaccine prices. The commercial vaccine manufacturers that license vaccines from the NVA would focus on efficient, high-volume manufacture at the lowest possible cost.

Monitoring and Evaluation

The NVA would rely on the combined expertise of AID, CDC, NIH, UNICEF, PAHO, WHO, and national governments to conduct CVI vaccine monitoring and evaluation. As noted in Chapter 6, the use and performance of existing CVI vaccines could be assessed and the need for new CVI products could be determined. All organizations with an interest in childhood vaccines would be involved in defining the requirements for new CVI products, as outlined above in the section Setting Priorities and Product Characterization.

Management and Organization

To be successful, the NVA would require a unified management structure with the authority and resources to undertake CVI product development. U.S. government agencies and the private sector could loan personnel to the NVA, perhaps on a rotating basis, as needed. The NVA could also be a focal point for training U.S. and overseas nationals in various aspects of vaccine development and manufacture.

Although the NVA would be a federal or federally supported entity, it would have to embody some characteristics not common to governmental organizations. For instance, it would need to be able to purchase supplies and equipment quickly, renovate facilities, and build new research laboratories and pilot production facilities. The NVA would need to have in-house regulatory expertise as well as staff experienced in negotiating issues related to intellectual property rights. In addition, it may be appropriate in some cases to limit the liability exposure of the NVA's manufacturing partners from claims of vaccine-related injury. The NVA must be able to hire staff at competitive salaries, license technology, and retain revenues from vaccine-product sales or licensing. One strategy may be to contract out the operation of the NVA pilot facility to the private sector—a so-called GOCO, a government-owned, contractor-operated entity. Although the NVA would not be expected to become entirely self-supporting, it is reasonable to expect that over time some NVA-related costs would be recovered. Although the NVA would have several entrepreneurial characteristics, it is crucial that it not fall prey to the very market forces that to date have prohibited the development of CVI vaccines. The governance of the NVA should be carefully considered to maximize its public health mission and entrepreneurial needs. Having a board of directors drawn from the public health community, government agencies, developing countries, academia, and the private sector could ensure that the NVA would not depart from its mission.

The NVA must be organized in a way that enables it to work in partnership with commercial manufacturers. Appropriate partnerships for vaccine development, large-scale manufacturing, or marketing and distribution will be essential to making new vaccines available at an accelerated pace.

Funding

The creation of new facilities or the expansion of existing vaccine development capacities to accommodate the NVA would require substantial public funding (Table 7-1). The committee estimates that the up-front capital expense of establishing the NVA would range from $30 million to

$75 million. The actual cost will depend on whether existing public-sector vaccine research and manufacturing capabilities are expanded or a new, freestanding unit is constructed and staffed. The proposed facilities should include applied research laboratories; pilot production capabilities for bacterial, viral, and parasitic vaccines (both at the bench-level scale and at a scale required to prepare sufficient amounts of vaccines for clinical trials); a sterile filling capacity; a quality control laboratory and quality assurance; and animal facilities. In addition, the facilities should be designed to permit different vaccines to be made. Each year, the NVA would spend between $25 million and $45 million on grants, contracts, and cooperative agreements to support its goals. Assuming annual operating costs and administrative services of $150,000 to $200,000 per person and a complement of 150 to 200 full-time staff (including contract officers; scientific R&D staff; program officers, regulatory affairs liaison, quality control, legal affairs, and administrative staff and facilities management personnel), the annual operating budget would total $30 million. Overall, the annual recurring costs would be between $55 million and $75 million. Additional funds would need to be provided for vaccine procurement guarantees.

TABLE 7-1 Estimated Costs of the Federal Vaccine Authority

Item	Cost (millions of $)
Capital costs	
Refurbishing an existing R&D and pilot facility	5–7
Construction of a new R&D and pilot facility	10–15
Equipment[a]	25–60
Total capital costs	30–75
Operating costs	
Contract and grants[b]	25–45
Annual operating expenses[c]	30
(Assume $150,000 x 200 people)	
Total operating costs	55–75

[a] Equipment includes that needed for R&D and a facility that manufactures pilot lots of vaccine under current Good Manufacturing Practices, and quality control and quality assurance.

[b] Assuming that funding of contract and grants would be parallel or greater than what the U.S. government currently spends on children's vaccine-related R&D, but less than most agency budgets for human immunodeficiency virus-related research.

[c] Assuming that operating expenses are estimated using a modified Delphi process. Estimated staff required includes those for research, pilot production laboratories, quality control and quality assurance, regulatory and legal affairs, and administrative services.

Location

The committee spent a considerable amount of time discussing where a new entity charged with developing CVI vaccine products might be located.Over the course of these deliberations, it became clear that there were a number of existing agencies that might serve as a home to such an organization. It is also possible, the committee realized, that the NVA should be placed in a quasigovernmental or entirely independent setting.

Points to Consider for Locating the CVI in an Existing Federal Agency

In the process of discussing these various possibilities, there emerged a number of "points to consider" that define what the committee felt to be important characteristics of any potential home for the NVA. Each agency considered by the committee meets some of these criteria; none satisfies all of them, however.

Rather than recommend a specific site for the new entity, the committee has decided to define some preliminary points to consider for locating the NVA (see the box "Points to Consider for Locating the NVA in an Existing Federal Agency"). The panel hopes that those charged with implementing its recommendations will use these points to consider when evaluating an appropriate location for the NVA. To assist in this process, the committee has tried to gauge how each of the agencies "fits" some of these criteria. Weighed against the points, each agency has pluses and minuses. Some of these are discussed below.

Options

U.S. Agency for International Development The U.S. Agency for International Development commits substantial resources to the support of immunization programs and vaccine-related research around the world. The agency is a funding entity and does not directly carry out activities itself. Thus, if it were to be given the responsibility for overseeing the NVA, it would need either to provide funding to an existing entity or to create a new operational unit.

There are precedents for this at AID. For example, many years ago the agency created Family Health International (FHI) to carry out primarily clinical contraceptive research. The Contraceptive Research and Development Program (CONRAD), a program administered by the University of Virginia, conducts research at earlier stages of development that

---

**Points to Consider for Locating the NVA
in an Existing Federal Agency**

• Correlation of the agency's mission to the mission of the NVA, particularly with regard to providing childhood vaccines to the developing world
• Intellectual and corporate culture and history
• Track record in developing and procuring vaccines
• Willingness to participate in CVI
• Avoidance of conflict of interest

---

complements the work of FHI. Together, FHI and CONRAD have many collaborative projects with private industry and conduct studies throughout the world. They have also undertaken technology transfer projects and have been active in regulatory, quality assurance, and quality control issues.

AID's direct involvement in the support of EPI programs, and its recent interest in CVI projects, means that it can provide a critical role in setting priorities. In addition, AID has been a major supporter of research on a malaria vaccine, a potential CVI product. AID could help to ensure the close coordination of U.S. vaccine-related activities with the programs of the global CVI.

Centers for Disease Control and Prevention The Centers for Disease Control and Prevention plays a vital role in purchasing and distributing vaccines in the United States and in assisting states with planning and implementing their own immunization programs. CDC also has considerable expertise in disease surveillance. The agency has established relationships with the health ministries of a number of foreign countries.

CDC conducts in-house vaccine-related R&D, much of it related to infectious diseases, and has a number of vaccine-related CRADAs with private industry. CDC has extensive experience in epidemiological surveillance, public health and disease prevention activities, and negotiating with commercial manufacturers for the purchase of vaccines.

U.S. Department of Defense The U.S. Department of Defense (Army) has an integrated and successful vaccine development program that is already working on CVI vaccines for use in military personnel. The department's vaccine program is product development oriented and has a successful track record getting vaccine products developed, licensed, and utilized. DOD has contributed to the development of a number of U.S.-licensed vaccines, including those against meningococcal disease and typhoid fever, which are of use to the CVI. Among DOD vaccines in clinical trials are those against shigella, cholera, dengue, malaria, and human immunodeficiency virus. DOD has considerable experience in working with the private sector, with both development-stage firms and commercial vaccine manufacturers. DOD has some experience in technology transfer overseas, but limited experience in facilitating the local production of vaccines. There are six DOD field laboratories around the world, each of which has the capacity to conduct and evaluate the results of vaccine field trials.

DOD might fear that an expanded mission in vaccine development would divert resources from its primary mission: protecting U.S. military personnel. In addition, there could be concerns overseas, however unfounded, about vaccines developed by the U.S. military.

U.S. Food and Drug Administration The U.S. Food and Drug Administration, through the Center for Biologics Evaluation and Research, is responsible for the scientific review of license applications for new biologics, including vaccines. FDA has unmatched expertise in the regulatory aspects of vaccine development. FDA has many years of experience in operating a successful in-house R&D program. Many of the studies which provided the basis for the development of the acellular pertussis vaccine were conducted in CBER laboratories. In addition, the agency has worked for many years to train foreign nationals in its laboratories, and FDA personnel participate actively in international consultations and in scientific committees at the WHO.

There is the potential for conflict of interest if the new entity were housed at the FDA, since the agency would be reviewing the regulatory compliance of the same products it was developing.

National Institutes of Health The National Institutes of Health, primarily through the National Institute of Allergy and Infectious Diseases, is the largest source of publicly funded vaccine research in the United States. NIH supports an extensive intramural research program and a larger program of extramural grants and contracts. Currently, NIH plans, encourages and supports CVI-related vaccine R&D. NIH has ties to overseas health and research organizations, and a number of investigators work informally with international colleagues. It also has limited capacity, primarily through contracts, to make small pilot lots of vaccine suitable for early-phase clinical testing.

Inasmuch as CVI-related activities benefit U.S. citizens, the missions of NIH and NVA are complementary. As currently authorized, however, the

NIH mission does not accommodate a major international effort. NIH's recent history has included efforts (through CRADAs, primarily) to reach out to and work with industry.

NIH has a distinguished intellectual history in the area of biomedical research, including vaccine-related R&D. NIH and its grantees have also had considerable success in the area of basic research related to vaccines. The agency's experience in product development is less extensive, but is growing particularly through the use of CRADAs and since the establishment of the vaccine evaluation units (see Chapter 6).

The National Vaccine Program The National Vaccine Program (NVP), located in the Office of the Assistant Secretary for Health (U.S. Public Health Service), is authorized to coordinate vaccine efforts in the United States. The NVP has no vaccine-related research or vaccine production capability. As authorized, the NVP was directed to develop and oversee the implementation of a National Vaccine Plan. Although the plan has not been released to the public, the concept of organizing and managing existing immunization resources in the United States is important and integral to the mission and functions of the NVA.

To accommodate an initiative of the size and scope of the NVA, the NVP would have to be authorized to become an operational entity (with a research laboratory and pilot production facility), and support for the NVP would have to be substantially increased. (Funding for the NVP fell from $9.5 million in 1991 to less than $3 million in 1993.) In addition, the stature of NVP would need to be elevated significantly.

Independent Organization In the past, the federal government has found it useful to charter new entities, such as the Tennessee Valley Authority, that are not bound by traditional government bureaucracy but that are responsive to public needs (see Appendix D). Establishing the NVA in a quasigovernmental or independent organization would have several advantages.

A quasigovernmental home for the NVA would provide the new organization with much desired flexibility, including the ability to hire and fire at will, offer salaries competitive with those offered in the private sector, and purchase needed equipment with little bureaucratic delay. At the same time, the NVA would retain some of the benefits of being associated with the federal government, including regular appropriations and close linkages to other agencies with a role in the CVI. As a truly independent entity, the NVA would need to raise its own capital and would interact with the government like any other private organization. If the NVA were an independent or even a quasigovernmental organization, it would not benefit from 28 USC §1498, as discussed in the section Intellectual Property Rights and in Chapter 5, unless the U.S. government treated the organization as a contractor for the purposes of vaccine acquisition.

The Henry M. Jackson Foundation, established by the U.S. Congress in 1983 and housed at the Uniformed Services University of Health Sciences in Bethesda, Maryland, is one example of such an arrangement. The foundation is a federally chartered, nonprofit, nongovernmental organization authorized to receive federal and nonfederal funds. In return, it carries out medical research and educational activities and consults on a contract basis for public and private sponsors, often through cooperative agreements. Flexibility is vital to the foundation's strength–it can employ both federal and nonfederal employees, receive patents, and negotiate licenses.

* * *

Vaccines are among the most cost-effective public health interventions available. Efforts to strengthen U.S. and global vaccination efforts will be based on the development of new and improved vaccines. The committee forwards the recommendation for a National Vaccine Authority having recognized and struggled with the burden and discomfort that the proposal of creating a new entity brings, most particularly at a time of limited resources and given national efforts to decrease government spending. The committee believes strongly, however, that the need and rationale for an entity like the NVA are compelling. An entity such as the NVA would fulfill a critical public health need and has the potential to protect children around the world while building on and strengthening public- and private-sector partnerships in the United States. The creation of an NVA will, for the first time, ensure the feasibility of a coherent program of development and production of CVI vaccines within the context and mandate of the 1986 legislation (P.L. 99-660) authorizing the NVP and requesting the National Vaccine Plan. The committee believes that the NVA, through a dynamic partnership between the public and private sectors, will offer the United States a new tool for ensuring the availability of novel vaccines and vaccine-related technologies for use in immunization programs around the world and in the domestic public health arena. The creation of an NVA-administered development and procurement program for CVI vaccines could greatly reduce the barriers to entry into vaccine production that many new biotechnology firms now face. By providing a market "springboard," this program could support the growth of U.S. biotechnology firms, potentially contributing to expansion in sources of supply for other types of vaccine products, contributing to the growth of a U.S. biotechnology industry, and aiding in the bolstering of U.S. competitiveness in this important sector. In the committee's view, the United States can and should play a decisive role in achieving the vision of the Children's Vaccine Initiative.

NOTE

1. The development of the first meningococcal vaccine is a good example of how the DOD approaches vaccine development and how the committee anticipates the NVA to function. Outbreaks of meningococcal meningitis had been a major problem for the United States in the mobilization of troops overseas throughout the 20th century. But in 1963, sulfonamide-resistant strains of meningococci became widespread in military recruits in the United States. Isolation of infected personnel and easement of crowding did little to stem the epidemics. The Walter Reed Army Institute of Research (WRAIR) responded by developing a major vaccine research and development program for meningococcal meningitis, under the leadership of Malcolm Artenstein. Over the next 6 years, the WRAIR conducted pioneering work on Group A, B, and C meningocci with a number of partners, most particularly the Rockefeller University. The WRAIR group was able to demonstrate both the technical feasibility of the vaccine and preliminary vaccine efficacy. The DOD was then able to attract private industry to invest in the manufacture and production of the vaccine. The meningococcal A and C vaccine is currently manufactured by private firms and sold to the DOD for use in military personnel.

REFERENCES

Flamm KJ. 1988. Targeting the Computer. Brookings Institution. Washington, D.C.

Levin RC. 1982. The Semiconductor Industry. Government and Technical Progress: A Cross-Industry Analysis, Nelson RR, ed. New York: Pergamon.

Institute of Medicine. 1992. Emerging Infections. Washington, D.C.: National Academy Press.

Mowery DC, Steinmueller WE. 1991. Prospects for entry by developing countries into the global integrated circuit industry: lessons from the U.S., Japan, and the NIES. CCC Working paper #91-8. Center for Research in Management. University of California at Berkeley.

Appendixes

A

Relevant Intellectual Property Rights Law

PATENTS

The primary goal of the U.S. patent system is to advance technological and economic development by stimulating innovation and investment. Patents serve two policy objectives: (1) By requiring disclosure of the manner and process of manufacturing an invention, the system encourages public disclosure of otherwise confidential information so that others are able to utilize it; and (2) by rewarding successful endeavors, patents provide inventors and their patrons with incentives to invest time and resources in research and development (Office of Technology Assessment, 1991).

Rights and Limitations

The protection granted under patent laws is a 17-year "right to exclude others from making, using, or selling the invention throughout the United States" (35 USC § 154 (Supp. 1982)). In return for that right, the patentee is required to disclose, in detail, the subject matter of the invention. Disclosure not only promotes additional research and development but also discourages unnecessary duplication of research. Disclosure is made in one's application for a patent, which contains a description of the invention and the specific inventive "claims" that one is seeking to patent. The level of detail disclosed in a patent application must be sufficient to allow one skilled in the art to make and use the invention. The patentee is not granted the right to exclude others from using the information disclosed in the patent application to produce and patent a noninfringing, new, different, and better product or process, as long as the new product or process meets the standard patent requirements.

It is important to note that the patent owner receives no affirmative right to make, use, or sell the claimed invention. In fact, a patent owner may find that practicing the invention infringes upon another party's previously issued patent. In that case, a patent owner must be authorized by the holder of the previously issued patent to use the owner's invention. For example, if a patentable improvement were made on a patented vaccine, the inventor of the improvement would need permission from the first-generation patent holder of the vaccine to make, use, or sell the improved vaccine.

There is no requirement that one use or license a patented invention, nor would one lose a U.S. patent for failing to use it. In contrast, most other countries impose a requirement that a patent owner must use or license a patented invention within a defined period of time. If patent protection is desired in a country other than the United States, one must apply for a patent in that country.

There is an exception to the general term of 17 years that is relevant to vaccines: When a patent claims that a human drug product, medical device, or food additive has undergone regulatory review for the product, device, or additive to be commercialized or marketed, the patent may be eligible for an extension of up to 5 years, if certain conditions are satisfied (Office of Technology Assessment, 1991). This exception is applied regularly to pharmaceutical products.

Infringement

One who violates the patent owner's rights is liable for patent infringement. If patent rights have indeed been violated, the owner is entitled to an injunction—a court order that prohibits an infringer from continuing to make, use, or sell the invention. The issuance of injunctive relief is within the discretion of the court. The Patent Act also authorizes an award of "damages adequate to compensate for the infringement, but in no event less than a reasonable royalty for the use made of the invention by the infringer" (USC 35 § 284). The method of calculating the damages award is within the discretion of the trial court. The court may increase the damages awarded by as much as threefold and may award interest and costs. This is usually done when the infringement was willful. The monetary loss suffered is assessed by comparing the patent owner's financial condition after the infringement occurs with what the condition would have been had the infringement not occurred. Actual damages should represent the monetary loss resulting from the infringement. If the patentee is unable to establish actual financial loss, damages are measured either by the gains/profits made by the infringer or by the "reasonable royalty" standard, which is the amount that one would have paid the patent owner for a license to use the invention.

Potential Barriers and Incentives

First-to-File Versus First-to-Invent

In the United States, when more than one patent application claiming the same invention is filed, the patent is awarded to the applicant who is able to establish that he/she was the first to conceive the invention and reduce it to practice. Applicants can submit a date of invention that is before the filing date. In contrast, nearly all other countries have laws whereby patent rights are awarded according to the earliest effective filing date of a patent application. The question of whether the United States should change its patent laws to conform to those of the rest of world has been a long-standing issue in discussions on patent law reform.

An Advisory Commission of Patent Law Reform was established in 1990 to advise the Secretary of Commerce on the need for reforms in the U.S. patent system. In August 1992, the commission put forth several recommendations, one of which was to convert the system in the United States from a first-to-invent to a first-to-file patent system. Among the points that the commission raised in citing the potential disadvantages of a first-to-file system were that (1) smaller companies might be at a disadvantage because of limited legal and financial resources and, therefore, would likely lose the "race to the Patent and Trademark Office" (PTO); (2) the PTO could be burdened with an increased volume of applications filed simply for defensive reasons; and (3) the exploration of commercialization opportunities prior to filing might be reduced because of the importance of early filing.

However, the commission felt that the advantages in changing to a first-to-file system would outweigh any negative effects and that first-to-file is a necessary component of any global intellectual property rights harmonization package (many other nations will not consider an intellectual property rights treaty unless the United States agrees to a first-to-file system). The benefits of a first-to-file system that the commission saw include the following: (1) it would encourage early filing, thereby promoting earlier disclosure of inventions and commercialization of products; (2) an agreement by the

United States to a global harmonization treaty could bring improvements in the patent protections offered by foreign countries for U.S. applicants seeking patents abroad; and (3) there would be a decrease in the complexities, time frame, and resources now associated with procedures devoted purely to determining who invented the product first.

To offset the potential disadvantages of a first-to-file system, the commission endorsed the change with three conditions: (1) the establishment of a provisional application procedure to expedite early filing at a reduced cost; (2) a grace period during which public disclosure of an invention would not affect patentability if an application is filed within 12 months of disclosure; and (3) "a third party who uses or makes substantial preparation for the use of invention before the filing date of an application on which patent is granted to another, has a right to continue to use the product under certain conditions" (Advisory Commission on Patent Law Reform, 1992, p. 21).

Other commission recommendations included extending the general patent term from 17 to 20 years (from the filing date) and that PTO funding should be maintained at a level that equips it to generally support an 18-month pendency period (Advisory Commission on Patent Law Reform, 1992).

Backlog in the Patent and Trademark Office

Over the past decade, the PTO has had to face sharply increasing numbers of biotechnology patent applications. From 1983 to 1988, the number of biotechnology applications rose 20 percent (applications in all other areas rose an average of 2.9 percent). To deal with this major influx, the PTO established an examining unit specifically for biotechnology in 1989. However, recent congressional reports reveal that the pendency period for biotechnology patent applications remains longer than that for any other technology (average pendency is 36.1 months for biotechnology patents compared with an average of 21 months for all other patents issued). Applications specifically related to immunology have an average pendency period of 44.1 months (Office of Technology Assessment, 1991). Nevertheless, it is important to note that patents (even those relating to biotechnology) are granted faster in the United States than in any major examining office in world, and by a significant amount of time (Office of Technology Assessment, 1991).

The reasons behind the backlog include the fact that the level of scientific scrutiny required to process an application for a biotechnology patent far exceeds that required for patents in most other areas. In addition, although the PTO has increased the number of biotechnology examiners (from 43 in 1986 to 140 in 1991) (Marshall, 1991), there has been a lack of success in retaining staff that are well-trained in biotechnology, because they are often successfully lured to private industry. Recently, the Industrial Biotechnology Association helped set up a Biotechnology Institute to educate PTO staff and improve the quality of their patent examinations.

The backlog has both positive and negative implications for industry. Long delays increase the uncertainty factor for potential patent holders because they are not privy to the contents of their competitors' applications, and the backlog of knowledge creates large volumes of "hidden knowledge" that may later become prior art. As a result, an inventor may file an application and discover much later that the application will be rejected because a previously filed application made the same claims.

Despite this problem, the backlog does present a potential advantage for products that require prolonged regulatory approval time. In these cases, a delay in obtaining a patent would extend the period of patent protection, since the 17-year term does not commence until the patent is actually issued (Office of Technology Assessment, 1991). Lengthy approval times are common in the vaccine industry.

Costs

One of the most serious problems facing patent seekers is the financial clout necessary to obtain and retain patents. The financial strain includes the legal, user, and maintenance fees paid to receive and keep a patent; however, the main monetary threat comes from the costs of litigation in cases of patent infringement. This threat presents a formidable budget item for smaller companies and universities, which often have limited resources. In most fields, the cost of obtaining a U.S. patent runs between $3,000 and $6,000. Biotechnology patents generally cost between $8,000 and $15,000 (the difference is a result of the extra time and examiners required) (Office of Technology Assessment, 1991).

Disclosure to Government Agencies

Several governmental or quasigovernmental entities regulate biotechnology research (most of these agencies are on the federal level). They require advance notice of all research proposed to be performed within their jurisdiction and assert the right to approve such research. This process typically requires the applicant to disclose with specificity the nature, scope, and purpose of the research. Often, however, this is precisely the information that the company performing the research wishes not to disclose and would rather maintain as a trade secret (Epstein, 1991).

Relevant Legislation and Terminology

Drug Price Competition and Patent Term Restoration Act of 1984 (P.L. 98-417)

One of the main purposes of this act was to restore part of the patent life lost during the regulatory approval process. It allows extension of the patent term, but not beyond 14 years of effective patent life. The actual extension granted is equal to the total time taken by the U.S. Food and Drug Administration (FDA) to review the new drug application plus one-half of the clinical testing time. Also, the act modified the abbreviated new drug application (ANDA) process to make FDA approval possible for marketing drugs that are equivalent to those approved by the FDA since 1962. Prior to the act, no drug approved after 1962 was available to a generic drug company for production, because the data provided to the FDA were treated as proprietary information. The new procedure permitted drug companies to submit bioequivalency data rather than repeating the safety and efficacy testing performed in connection with a manufacturer's prior new drug application (Miller and D'Angelo, 1989). Vaccines, however, are currently excluded from the ANDA process.

Omnibus Trade and Competitiveness Act (P.L. 100-418)

This act states that if anyone imports into, sells, or uses within the United States a product made using a U.S.-patented process, he/she is liable as an infringer (if the activity occurs during the patent term). Prior to this act, no monetary damages could be obtained as a result of the action described above, and the U.S. manufacturer had to show injury to an established domestic industry to get an injunction. The act also provides the U.S. patent holder with access to federal courts, in addition to the International Trade Commission, as a means of enforcement action (Office of Technology Assessment, 1991).

Grace Period

Currently, the United States gives the inventor who publishes patentable information, or who uses the invention commercially before filing a patent application, a 1-year grace period to file the patent application. This is especially advantageous for smaller companies and individual scientists who might feel the need to publish research findings as soon as possible (Office of Technology Assessment, 1991).

Orphan Drug Act of 1983 (P.L. 99-91)

The Orphan Drug Act offers incentives to invest in products that, because of a smaller market for the products, are not likely to offer an adequate return on investment to the company. The government offers grants, tax breaks, and most importantly, 7 years of market exclusivity to the first manufacturer to gain the FDA's approval for a product designated as an orphan drug.

Patent and Trademark Amendments of 1980 (P.L. 96-517)

The U.S. Congress passed these amendments in order to promote a uniform patent policy that would foster cooperative agreements and commercialize government-funded inventions. The law permits nonprofit entities (including universities) and small businesses to retain the titles to patents resulting from federally funded research, with the federal agency retaining a worldwide, nonexclusive license. The law, which gave statutory preferences to small businesses and nonprofit organizations, was extended to larger companies in 1983 (Office of Technology Assessment, 1991).

Experimental Use Exception

Added as an amendment to the Drug Price Competition and Patent Term Restoration Act of 1984, this clause provides an exception to infringement on patent rights, whereby it is not an act of infringement to "make, use or sell a patented invention solely for uses reasonably related to the development and submission of information under a Federal law which regulates the manufacture, use or sale of drugs" (Epstein, 1991, p. 452.14). For example, it would not be an infringement to use another party's patented vaccine to collect data that may be required in order to obtain FDA approval for one's own vaccine.

TRADE SECRETS (KNOW-HOW)

Trade secrets make up an area of intellectual property law that provides an effective and efficient method of protecting commercially sensitive and important business information. For vaccines, issues relating to "know-how" are equally important as the patent concerns discussed above.

Definition

A trade secret consists of any type of material or information that is valuable, not generally known publicly, and kept secret. There are no subject matter limitations on what can constitute a trade secret; therefore, a broad array of information can be protected as such, including scientific processes such as the know-how to make vaccines, other biologics, and pharmaceuticals.

Secrecy is the most important criterion that the information must meet to be a trade secret. However, the law recognizes that for a trade secret to be commercially utilized, it must often be disclosed to other parties, including customers, employees, licensees, coventurers, and suppliers. Consequently, only relative secrecy, or a reasonable element of secrecy, must exist.

Confidentiality

A trade secret cannot be known by the public or widely known by other companies. In addition, even if the information is not actually known by others, trade secret status is lost if the information is available for others to obtain and learn. Thus, the information cannot be published or distributed in any manner. If the trade secret is disclosed by the product itself, the product must remain confidential.

If a company believes that it has a trade secret, the company is required by law to protect the information's confidentiality. In the context of licensing, this means that any exchange of trade secret information must be protected by a nondisclosure agreement that rigorously protects the confidentiality of the trade secret, not only during the term of the license but also after expiration or termination of the license agreement.

Rights of the Trade Secret Owner

The owner of a trade secret possesses legal rights that prevent the unauthorized disclosure and/or use of the trade secret by other parties. In certain circumstances, these rights can be asserted absent a contractual agreement with the individual or corporation whose unauthorized disclosure and/or use is sought to be prevented.

Rights Against Individuals in Privity

In order to exploit trade secrets commercially, the secrets will probably be disclosed by the trade secret owner. In making this disclosure, however, the trade secret owner will want to preserve any rights arising by virtue of trade secret ownership–in particular, the right to prevent subsequent unauthorized disclosure and/or use of the information. The two methods by which the owner can maintain this right are protection by contract and protection by an implied contract/special relationship.

Protection by Contract The owner may protect the trade secret information from unauthorized disclosure and/or use by entering into a contract–termed a *nondisclosure* or *confidentiality agreement*–with all licensees or other individuals to whom the owner discloses the trade secret. In the event of an unauthorized disclosure and/or use, the trade secret owner can sue for breach of contract and seek an injunction to prevent future unauthorized disclosure and/or use, as well as monetary damages for past unauthorized disclosure and/or use.

Implied Contract/Special Relationships In certain circumstances, a trade secret owner has the right to prevent the unauthorized disclosure and/or use of trade secrets because of an implied contract or special relationship with the person to whom the owner disclosed trade secrets.

A licensor–licensee relationship, along with certain other relationships between the trade secret owner and another party, is deemed by the law as a "special relationship." When a trade secret is disclosed by its owners pursuant to a special relationship, the individual to whom the trade secret is disclosed has the duty to maintain the confidentiality of the trade secret and not to use it to the detriment of its owner. A trade secret owner can sue when this duty is breached, and as described above, the trade secret owner can seek an injunction and/or damages.

Rights Against Third Parties

A trade secret owner also wants to protect his/her trade secrets from the unauthorized disclosure and/or use by a third party—that is, a party to whom the trade secret owner did not directly disclose the information. This situation most frequently arises when an employee of the trade secret owner changes jobs and the former employer/trade secret owner wishes to prevent the new employer from disclosing and/or using the trade secrets that the employee learned during his/her prior employment.

A trade secret owner may assert a misappropriation claim against a third party to prevent or remedy unauthorized disclosure and/or use by a third party when the third party knows that the information is considered to be a trade secret and the information was disclosed to the third party through a breach of duty (either by virtue of a contract or by a special relationship/implied contract owed to the trade secret owner).

Additional Rights of a Trade Secret Owner

The owner of a trade secret also possesses the right to prevent individuals who learn the trade secret through improper means from disclosure and/or use of the information. According to the law, "improper means" includes obtaining another's trade secrets through (1) illegal activities, (2) fraud and misrepresentation, and (3) legal but improper means, such as industrial espionage or other extraordinary measures.

Rights to Use Another's Trade Secrets

A party can learn, obtain, and use another's trade secret in three lawful ways. First, a party may independently discover another's trade secret; trade secret law does not give a trade secret owner rights against one who learns the secret through independent invention. Second, a party may properly "reverse engineer" a trade secret in order to learn it. Finally, a party can learn and use another's trade secret through a disclosure to it which is not in breach of a contract or special relationship or with knowledge of such a breach.

REFERENCES

Advisory Commission on Patent Law Reform. 1992. A Report to the Secretary of Commerce. August. Washington, D.C.

Epstein MA. 1991. Modern Intellectual Property. Englewood Cliffs, New Jersey: Prentice-Hall Law and Business.

Marshall E. 1991. The patent game: Raising the ante. Science 253:20–24.

Miller CE, D'Angelo M. 1989. Patents, price and patient interest. Chemtech. March. Pp. 156–159.

Office of Technology Assessment. 1991. Biotechnology in a Global Economy. Washington, D.C.

B

National Vaccine Injury Compensation Program

DEFINITION AND PURPOSE

The National Vaccine Injury Compensation Program (NVICP) is the first-ever U.S. "no-fault" compensation system for patients (or their families) who suffer serious adverse reactions from required childhood vaccines. By removing most of the liability burden from manufacturers for immunization-related injuries, the program was expected to help stabilize the supply and price of vaccines (Mariner, 1991). The NVICP was established as part of the 1986 National Childhood Vaccine Injury Act (Public Health Service Act, 1987; 100 Stat. 3756, codified as Title XXI of the Public Health Service Act at 42 USC 300aa-1 *et seq.* (Supp. V 1987)), but it did not become operational until the fall of 1988.

BACKGROUND

The NVICP is the result of nearly two decades of controversy over whether and how adverse reactions to childhood vaccines should be addressed. Before the program became law, the sole recourse for parents who felt that their children had been harmed by a vaccine was to sue the vaccine manufacturer–an expensive and time-consuming process (Mariner, 1991).

In 1982, news stories began to describe the plight of children with adverse reactions to vaccines (Mazzuca, 1992; WRC-TV, 1982). Vaccine manufacturers were confronted by claims for disabilities believed to be caused by immunization. Some feared damage awards of several million dollar cases, as there were no reliable guidelines for predicting the limits and the magnitude of liability litigation. Some companies saw the threat of huge settlements as an unreasonable risk, particularly given the development costs and relatively low profit margin associated with vaccines. A fair number of companies simply dropped out of the vaccine manufacturing business altogether, many citing liability (U.S. Congress, House, 1986). Those companies that remained in the market began to raise their prices significantly, in part to cover anticipated liability expenses (Institute of Medicine, 1985).

In the early to mid-1980s, several committees, including the Institute of Medicine Committee on Vaccine Supply and Innovation (Institute of Medicine, 1985), endorsed the creation of a no-fault compensation system. In 1984, the American Academy of Pediatrics took the initiative in seeking federal legislation to create a national compensation program. Several bills were introduced by members of Congress and were debated in congressional hearings, and in 1986, the National Vaccine Injury Compensation Program was enacted under the sponsorship of Representative Henry Waxman and Senator Orrin Hatch.

FILING A CLAIM UNDER NVICP

In the first step in the claims process, the petitioner files a petition with the U.S. Claims Court to demonstrate eligibility. A randomly assigned special master then reviews the petition, elicits a recommendation from the NVICP Office in the Department of Health and Human Services, and makes a determination regarding eligibility (all special masters are lawyers, almost always with no prior experience in vaccines). The Secretary of the Department of Health and Human Services is the respondent in the proceedings and may contest the petitioner's claim. If the petitioner is eligible for the program, the special master then decides the amount of compensation. Neither vaccine manufacturers nor healthcare providers are part of this process, and there are no determinations of legal fault. Once accepted into the program, petitioners are prohibited from bringing civil action for damages until after a decision is made.

There are two types of claimants: retrospective and prospective. Retrospective petitioners are those injured before October 1, 1988, who were required to file by January 31, 1991. Congress appropriated $80 million per year for the first 4 years of the program to pay retrospective claims. Prospective petitioners are those who were injured on or after October 1, 1988. They are required to file within 2 to 4 years of the date of the claimed injury. Funds for awards to prospective petitioners are taken from the compensation trust fund supported by an excise tax on vaccines. (As of January 1, 1993, this tax had not been reauthorized by the Congress.)

If appropriations are insufficient to permit payment of any award, the petitioner is exempt from the prohibition against bringing a civil lawsuit. There is also a cap of 3,500 on the number of retrospective petitioners who may be compensated under the program. A total of 4,069 pre-1988 claims were filed, but only 1,290 of these had been adjudicated by February 1993. A total of 641 claimants had been awarded a total of $297.2 million. The number of post-1988 vaccine injury cases in the system has continued to increase, from only 1 in 1989, to 31 in 1990, 119 in 1991, and 191 in 1992. As of February 1993, 64 post-1988 claimants had been awarded a total of $26.5 million. Of the 1,405 retrospective and prospective claims that had been adjudicated by February 1993, the majority were dismissed (790 claims), and 156 were deemed not compensable (National Vaccine Injury Compensation Program, 1993).

Compensation amounts are calculated by taking into account nonreimbursable medical and related expenses, lost earnings, and pain and suffering. In cases of death, a fixed sum of $250,000 is awarded. The average award for a pre-1988 case is $1 million (National Vaccine Injury and Compensation Program, 1993). Since the program is an alternative, rather than an exclusive, source of compensation, each petitioner has the option to reject the decision made on the petition. However, petitioners in prospective cases are not allowed to begin a lawsuit until they have filed a claim with the program, received a final judgment, and rejected it in favor of litigation (retrospective petitioners had the option of staying with their lawsuit or dropping it in order to file a claim with the program).

Petitioners have two levels of appeal if they are not satisfied with the special master's decision. They can request that the U.S. Claims Court review the decision; if, after this is done, the petitioner is still not satisfied, he/she may appeal to the U.S. Court of Appeals.

KEY CHARACTERISTICS

For the NVICP to serve as an effective option to litigation, the compensation process must work quickly. In order to expedite matters, the program does not involve itself with causation, one of the most costly and time-consuming components of a tort action for personal injury. Things have not moved nearly as rapidly as was hoped, however. For retrospective cases filed after December 1989, decisions were to have been made within 240 days; because of heavy case loads, Congress extended this "suspension time" to 780 days. For post-1988 cases, the processing time is approximately

12 to 15 months (National Vaccine Injury Compensation Program, 1992). Causation is presumed for conditions listed in the program's Vaccine Injury Table. The table lists illnesses, disabilities, injuries, and conditions covered by the program. If the conditions of the petitioner are not included in the table, they must then prove causation by a covered vaccine. Although the overall utility of the table has been widely accepted, there are several problems with it. For example, there have been a number of disputes over some listed conditions, as well as difficulties in defining "acceptable evidence" for the conditions. By the end of March 1990, the Division of Vaccine Injury Compensation of the U.S. Department of Health and Human Services had recommended against compensating 74 percent of 57 petitions on the grounds that the injury did not fit the table. However, the court awarded compensation for 90 percent of those 57 petitions, rejecting most of the division's recommendations (Mariner, 1992). The Department of Health and Human Services is developing proposed regulations to amend the table, based in part on the 1991 Institute of Medicine report entitled *Adverse Effects of Pertussis and Rubella Vaccines.*

REFERENCES

Institute of Medicine. 1985. Vaccine Supply and Innovation. Washington, D.C.: National Academy Press.

Mariner WK. 1991. Innovation and Challenge: The First Year of the National Vaccine Injury Compensation Program. Prepared for the Administrative Conference of the United States. May. Washington, D.C.

Mariner WK. 1992. Update: The National Vaccine Injury Compensation Program. Health Affairs 11:255-265.

Mazzuca L. 1992. Shot through with problems. Business Insurance. August 24. p. 1.

National Vaccine Injury Compensation Program. 1992. Analysis of Vaccine Excise Tax Levels–Update. Rockville, Maryland: Health Resources and Services Administration.

National Vaccine Injury Compensation Program. 1993. Weekly Status Report, February 22. Rockville, Maryland: Health Resources and Services Administration.

U.S. Congress, House. 1986. Childhood Immunizations. A report prepared by the Subcommittee on Health and the Environment, Committee on Energy and Commerce. September. Washington, D.C.

WRC-TV. 1982. DPT vaccine roulette. Videorecording. Washington, D.C.

C

Regulatory Aspects of Vaccine Development, Manufacture, and Distribution

Regulatory issues are involved in nearly every aspect of vaccine development, manufacturing, and marketing approval. Regulations come into play from the time of vaccine design and clinical testing, through manufacturing, to when the final product is distributed for widespread use.

Section 351 of the Public Health Service Act (P.L. 78-410) requires a manufacturer of biological products to first obtain a license to ship the product (vaccine) in interstate and/or foreign commerce or to import the vaccine into the United States. To obtain a license, manufacturers must make a vaccine by an approved procedure, in approved facilities, and by an approved staff. Standards and requirements for vaccine licensure in the United States are generated and enforced by the Center for Biologics Evaluation and Research (CBER) at the U.S. Food and Drug Administration (FDA). The licensing regulations are published in the Code of Federal Regulations, Title 21, Part 600.

THE LICENSURE PROCESS

The process of obtaining a license to manufacture and distribute a vaccine is complex and time-consuming, both for the manufacturer and the FDA. To obtain permission to conduct a clinical study, the sponsor must have first prepared pilot lots for experimental purposes including preclinical

164

testing in animals. When the pilot lots are ready for clinical testing in humans, the sponsor submits a Notice of Claimed Investigational Exemption for a New Drug; from that point on, the product is referred to as an investigational new drug (IND). A complete IND application includes (1) descriptions of the composition, source, and manufacturing process of the product; (2) quality control and the methods used to test the vaccine's safety, purity, and potency; (3) a summary of all laboratory and preclinical animal testing; (4) a detailed description of the proposed clinical study; and (5) names and qualifications of each clinical investigator. During a 30-day waiting period, the IND application is reviewed by the FDA to determine whether human subjects will be exposed to unwarranted risks (Hopps et al., 1988).

Although an establishment license (described below in more detail) is not required to begin a clinical trial, it is important that the manufacturer produces vaccine lots in a facility meeting current Good Manufacturing Practices. Plants that follow current Good Manufacturing Practices must demonstrate complete control over product components, equipment, manufacturing environment, record-keeping, and personnel. There should be no changes in the facility or manufacturing process that could alter any critical aspects of the product between the time that pivotal lots for clinical trials are prepared to establish vaccine efficacy and the time that lots are prepared for final licensing and distribution (Weber, 1991).

If the manufacturer is convinced that the vaccine is safe and effective after having performed clinical trials, an application for a license is made to CBER. The Product License Application (PLA) is an exhaustive document which includes (1) a detailed description of the manufacturing procedures, testing methods, and process controls for the product; (2) results of all laboratory tests performed on a specified number of lots (including stability testing); (3) results of clinical studies; and (4) proposed labeling (Hopps et al., 1988).

The newly created Office of Vaccines Research and Review within CBER is now responsible for the review of vaccine IND applications and PLAs. The internal review process entails a detailed examination and analysis of the submitted data for scientific content and accuracy and for compliance with applicable regulations. Individuals from other offices of CBER may also participate in the vaccine review and approval process.

The vaccine manufacturer must also submit an Establishment License Application (ELA). The ELA describes (1) the organization and personnel, (2) buildings and work areas, (3) equipment and systems, (4) control of components and containers, (5) production and process controls, (6) packaging and labeling controls, and (7) records and reports to be maintained (Hopps et al., 1988). The manufacturer must satisfy the FDA that it has complied with an extensive body of regulations termed Good Manufacturing Practices throughout the production process. Validation is a critical component of current Good Manufacturing Practices compliance. Essentially, validation is demonstrating that the manufacturing procedures, tests, equipment, and systems perform as intended and produce the expected and consistent results.

The Office of Establishment Licensing and Product Surveillance within CBER is responsible for the review of vaccine ELAs. The internal review consists primarily of determining that (1) the layout of the manufacturing facilities, the equipment, and the systems are adequate for vaccine production and storage; (2) the expert personnel have been properly trained for their assigned duties and functions; and (3) validation of the equipment, systems, and process controls is satisfactory.

FDA approval for licensure is based on (1) a satisfactory review of all data indicating that the product is safe and effective for its intended use; (2) review and acceptance of the manufacturer's labeling; (3) a satisfactory review of the manufacturer's protocols that summarize the manufacturing and testing on a specified number of vaccine lots to establish the consistency of the process; (4) confirmatory testing by CBER on product samples received from the manufacturer; and (5) a satisfactory FDA inspection of the manufacturer's vaccine production facilities (Hopps et al., 1988).

In November 1992, the FDA published guidelines on cooperative manufacturing for biological products, recognizing four types of manufacturing arrangements: short supply, divided, shared, and contract.

Short supply allows a licensed manufacturer to obtain from an unlicensed facility source materials that are declared to be in short supply. Historically, the short supply provisions are provided under an old FDA regulation that is rarely used today by licensed vaccine manufacturers. *Divided manufacturing* permits two manufacturers, each licensed to produce the biologic in its entirety, to produce such a product together. Approval of this arrangement requires both manufacturers to file PLA amendments that describe what procedures will be performed at each facility, along with copies of the labeling to be used for the intermediate and finished products. This arrangement is not often used by licensed vaccine manufacturers.

Under a *shared arrangement*, two or more manufacturers participate in the manufacture of a biological product, with each manufacturer required to hold both an establishment license and a product license for the ingredient that it contributes to the process. However, none of the manufacturers are required to be licensed to perform all steps in the manufacturing process. To qualify for licensure approval, each manufacturer performs significant steps in the manufacture of the active ingredient of the product. Under a shared arrangement, the manufacturer of the final product also has the ultimate responsibility for providing data that demonstrate the potency, safety, and effectiveness of the product. Licenses are not issued to any manufacturer until the final product has been shown to be safe and effective.

Under a *contract arrangement*, only one of the manufacturers holds a license, while the other performs one or more steps that would not be considered "significant" to warrant a license. Examples would include filling and labeling of final containers of the product. However, all steps of manufacturing performed at the unlicensed facility must be under the supervision and control of the licensed manufacturer. Contract arrangements are frequently used by biologics manufacturers, including vaccine manufacturers.

POSTLICENSING

Manufacture

After a manufacturer has obtained licensure, the vaccine is subject to lot-by-lot release by CBER. Samples and a summary of testing may be required for each lot presented for release at any time. The approved license application becomes the standard that a manufacturer must follow. Any departure from the approved procedure is a potential basis for regulatory action. During the life of a product, however, changes from the original methods may be necessary. In these cases, the FDA requires that no unauthorized change take place and that the manufacturer has an internal system in place through which proposed changes are reviewed and evaluated. All important changes must be reported to CBER 30 days in advance, and these changes in manufacturing procedures or in labeling may not be implemented until they are approved by CBER. Depending on the nature and extent of the change, CBER will make a determination of whether a new license application would be required or a license amendment to the PLA would suffice. Examples of changes requiring an amendment would be new dosage forms or modifications in the purification process, given that the integrity of the product remains unchanged. Similarly, modifications to manufacturing facilities or equipment would require the manufacturer to file an amendment to the approved ELA. In any case, the manufacturer must demonstrate on a regular basis that the vaccine meets stability requirements.

The shipment of licensed bulk vaccines for export is permitted by CBER, provided that the bulk vaccine is prepared in exactly the same way as specified in the manufacturer's approved PLA up to the point of shipment. Approval of bulk shipments requires the manufacturer to file a product license amendment (in addition to the PLA), describing at what step of manufacturing the bulk vaccine will be shipped, as well as the shipping and packaging controls and the labeling that will accompany the shipment. The labeling must specify that the bulk vaccine is "For Further Manufacturing Only." The license amendment must also include a written agreement, signed by the foreign consignee, stating that labeling of the finished filled containers of vaccine will not bear the U.S. license number of the bulk manufacturer nor make such reference in the labeling. Since U.S. Customs will detain a biological product from entering the country without a license number, the agreement effectively bars the product from being returned to the United States.

Distribution

A vaccine must be packaged to withstand the handling and storage to which it will be subjected in transit; therefore, the manufacturer must, as far as possible, control the route and shipment method. In addition, the manufacturer must maintain destination records of the vaccine, to initiate a rapid and efficient recall should it be necessary. Also, it is the manufacturer's responsibility to ensure that only approved labeling is used in any labeling or packaging operation (Weber, 1991). Finally, through the Vaccine Adverse Events Reporting System (see Chapter 6), the FDA, along with the Centers for Disease Control and Prevention, is responsible for monitoring adverse reactions to vaccines.

THE DRUG EXPORT AMENDMENTS ACT OF 1986

In addition to the export of vaccines under the licensing provisions of the Public Health Service Act, the Drug Export Amendments Act of 1986 (P.L. 99-660) permits the export of unlicensed biological products under certain specified conditions. The Drug Export Amendments establish three separate tracks for the export of unapproved drugs and unlicensed biological products. Under track 1, the FDA is authorized to approve the export of finished products that are not approved for marketing in the United States, but that have the same active ingredients as a product for which marketing approval is actively being sought in the United States. Export under track 1 is limited to 21 specified industrialized countries.

The FDA is also authorized to approve the export of drugs and biologics intended for the treatment of tropical diseases. Congress drafted this provision to enable the export of drugs and biologics intended for diseases and conditions in developing countries but that do not exist to a significant extent in the United States, and thus would not be likely candidates for market approval in the United States. Export approval permits for track 2 products are not limited to the 21 specified industrialized countries. Normally, the FDA anticipates that approval under track 2 would ordinarily be based on data from two well-controlled clinical trials, but that the trials would not necessarily have to meet the full detail and documentation requirements necessary for approval of a U.S. marketing application. However, there must be evidence that the product is safe and effective for the intended use in the country to which it is to be exported.

Finally, the act permits the FDA to approve the export of partially processed human biological products that are intended for further manufacture in one or more of the same set of 21 specified industrialized track 1 countries. These track 3 products must be approved, or be in the process of being approved, in the country of destination (U.S. Food and Drug Administration, 1990).

REFERENCES

Hopps HE, Meyer BC, Parkman PD. 1988. Regulation and testing of vaccines. Vaccines, Plotkin SA and Mortimer EA, eds. Philadelphia: W.B. Saunders Company.

U.S. Food and Drug Administration. 1990. A Review of FDA's Implementation of the Drug Export Amendments of 1986. Rockville, Maryland.

Weber JCW. 1991. Regulatory Aspects of Vaccine Development. Vaccines for Fertility Regulation, Ada GL and Griffin PD, eds. Cambridge: Cambridge University Press.

D

Strategies for Achieving Full U.S. Participation in the Children's Vaccine Initiative

The Institute of Medicine Committee on the Children's Vaccine Initiative recognized early on in its deliberations that achieving the vision of the Children's Vaccine Initiative (CVI) would require choosing among a range of strategies and options, each of which could have profound implications for the future development, production, delivery, and use of vaccines for children in economically disadvantaged countries of the world. To facilitate consideration of possible options, the committee devised three major "strategies." Each strategy depends on certain requirements and each has positive and negative implications. It should be noted that these strategies and the various approaches they encompass are not mutually exclusive. The following discussion of these strategies is designed to permit those with a commitment to childhood vaccines to evaluate a number of new ideas and approaches to achieving the goals of the CVI. In discussing and defining strategies as to how to enhance overall United States public- and private-sector participation in the CVI, the committee recognized the following:

- The combined scientific base of the U.S. public and private sectors for the development of vaccines is not exceeded anywhere in the world.
- The process of vaccine development, from basic research through to commercialization, breaks down for those vaccines of little commercial interest, most particularly at the point of pilot production.

170

• Without a major initiative in research, development, production, and procurement capability, new vaccines and new combinations will be used exclusively in economically advantaged countries, while less advantaged countries will remain dependent on the current Expanded Program on Immunization (EPI) vaccines and on the local production of vaccines.

• It is insufficient just to develop new and improved vaccines; such vaccines must be manufactured and made available to the CVI and EPI.

• U.S. pharmaceutical firms are profit-driven; their continued presence in vaccines depends on adequate returns on their investments.

• The availability of vaccines in the United States depends almost entirely on incentives to commercial firms to develop and produce them.

• Over 80 percent of the world's children are born in countries producing one or more of the EPI vaccines and almost 60 percent of diphtheria and tetanus toxoids and pertussis vaccine used in the world today is produced in the country that uses it.

• U.S. inner-city and rural populations face vaccine delivery and coverage problems similar to those being addressed by CVI, and many CVI goals are compatible with national interests.

STRATEGY 1: RETAIN THE CURRENT SYSTEM

It is entirely possible that the current vaccine system, which has many strengths, could be augmented sufficiently to permit full U.S. participation in the CVI. The process of vaccine innovation in the United States, involves numerous organizations in both the public and private sectors. In contrast, the actual production of vaccines depends on a handful of commercial and two state manufacturers.

Under the current system, commercial manufacturers pursue the development of vaccines for which there is perceived to be adequate returns on investment. For the most part, commercial vaccine manufacturers cannot justify their investment either in the development of new vaccines or in the improvement of existing vaccines intended for predominately developing-country markets. Some priority CVI vaccines have limited industrialized-country markets and are therefore perceived to be unprofitable. The two largest buyers of vaccines internationally, the Pan American Health Organization (PAHO) and the United Nations Children's Fund (UNICEF), have procured vaccines for many years at very low prices. Given that no new vaccines have been developed and introduced to the UNICEF/PAHO/EPI market since its inception, it would appear that the prices quoted to UNICEF/PAHO are not sufficient to stimulate vaccine innovation.

Within the current system, small and medium-sized biotechnology companies are a new force in the pharmaceutical industry, contributing especially to the development of new and improved technologies for constructing vaccines. Few of these companies, however, have the capability to manufacture a vaccine on a pilot scale, and almost none have a full-scale manufacturing facility. To manufacture their products on a commercial scale, most biotechnology companies must form strategic alliances with larger pharmaceutical companies. Ultimately, then, the decision to make a vaccine rests entirely with large, private industry, which bases its activities on the perception of a commercial market.

Assuming no fundamental changes in the current system of vaccine innovation summarized above, the committee identified three possible approaches for enhancing U.S. participation in the CVI: substantial increase in financial support for CVI vaccine research carried out by government agencies, federal purchase of existing vaccines for use in programs such as the EPI, and improvement in the delivery of existing vaccines.

Option 1: Increased Funding for CVI Vaccine Research

Under this option, substantial new funding would be added to the budgets of the various agencies involved in vaccine-related research. The additional money would supplement the investment in vaccine research at the National Institutes of Health (NIH), the U.S. Department of Defense (DOD), the U.S. Food and Drug Administration (FDA), and the Centers for Disease Control and Prevention (CDC).

The main benefit of this option is a continued commitment to vaccine research in the public sector. In addition, increased resources would be directed toward vaccines that are most relevant to the CVI. However, this option does not encourage enhanced participation by private industry, neither biotechnology firms nor established manufacturers, and the superb resources that they could bring to the CVI. In this sense, it does not foster optimal participation in the CVI by the United States. Also, by simply increasing funds for the beginning stages of vaccine development, this option does not effectively overcome any of the obstacles in the current system that might impede the process of vaccine development and manufacture, most particularly the shortage of facilities used to produce pilot lots of vaccine. Finally, injecting additional resources into public-sector vaccine research would do little to increase the commercial viability of CVI vaccines; as a result, production of these vaccines would be unlikely.

For this option to materialize, an estimate of resource requirements would need to be made and the U.S. Congress would have to appropriate the additional funds. No other major changes in the status quo would be required, except that the budgets, and possibly staffs, of certain government agencies would increase.

Contribution to the Global CVI

This option would contribute to the global CVI by maintaining a strong U.S. presence in basic and applied vaccine research. There would likely be substantial spin-offs to the global CVI for new approaches to vaccine development. Unfortunately, the global CVI lacks the capability to ensure that new approaches are tested and developed.

Option 2: Purchase Existing Vaccines

Under this option, the U.S. government, through the U.S. Agency for International Development (AID), could procure bulk or finished vaccines from U.S.-based manufacturers for use in immunization programs in developing countries. Another approach would be for the U.S. government to contribute money directly to UNICEF, enhancing UNICEF's ability to implement immunization activities, including the procurement and distribution of vaccines. (It is unlikely, however, that U.S. manufacturers would bid on UNICEF contracts [see Chapter 4]).

This option would enable the United States to contribute its high-quality vaccines to children in the developing world. In addition, AID could advance technology transfer to developing countries by supplying bulk vaccine, accompanied by assistance for training, quality control, and quality assurance in filling and packaging the vaccine. Lastly, the first two alternatives included in this option would guarantee an overseas market to U.S. manufacturers for existing vaccines or bulk products.

Despite these advantages, this option does not build upon U.S. strengths in vaccine research and development. The purchase of existing vaccines is unlikely to lead to the development of new CVI vaccines under current market arrangements. In addition, because this approach is resource intensive, it is not likely to be sustainable in the long term, particularly with the advent of more expensive combination vaccines. Furthermore, any benefit to countries receiving U.S.-purchased vaccines may be reduced if the value of those purchases is deducted from an overall U.S. foreign aid package.

The success of this option would depend on the ability of selected U.S. government agencies to alter the ways in which they operate. For instance, the Office of Health at AID would have to orient itself more toward procurement. In essence, the U.S. government, through AID, would be embarking on a price subsidy policy analogous to that in agriculture by buying vaccines at one price and selling them overseas at a lower price. This option would also require that international activities within the FDA be expanded in order to increase its assistance with quality control and quality assurance in developing countries.

Contribution to the Global CVI

This option would enhance the quality control capacity of developing countries that are or would be capable of manufacturing CVI vaccine products and would foster production-sharing between the United States and those developing countries. It might also enable the United States to supply CVI vaccines to developing countries; however, under this option these vaccines would most likely be developed only if they also served an industrialized-country market.

Option 3: Improve Vaccine Delivery

Under this option, U.S. foreign aid efforts would focus on enhancing vaccine delivery in the developing world. This could be done, for example, by strengthening health infrastructure. Implicit in this approach is the assumption that the best way for the United States to help alleviate problems of immunization coverage in the developing world is by improving the delivery of existing vaccines rather than contributing to the development and introduction of new vaccines.

This option would help to provide needed resources and supplies to achieve better immunization coverage in the developing world. However, a focus on vaccine delivery is not likely to result in the development of CVI vaccines, some of which would facilitate easier delivery by virtue of their characteristics. For example, heat-stable polio vaccine would reduce cold-chain difficulties, and combination or sustained-release vaccines would reduce the number of needed visits to health clinics. This option, then, would not capitalize on the significant U.S. resources devoted to vaccine research, development, and manufacture. Finally, technology transfer to developing countries would not be facilitated under this option.

To accommodate this new mission, AID would need to either shift more resources into vaccine delivery efforts or convince the U.S. Congress to appropriate new funds for this purpose. In other respects, current funding streams to U.S. government agencies would continue, although the United States would probably contribute additional amounts to UNICEF and PAHO for vaccine procurement.

Contribution to the Global CVI

This scenario would channel additional U.S. resources into enhancing the delivery of existing vaccines rather than ensuring the development and supply of new and improved vaccines. As a result, the burden of developing CVI vaccines would rest within the international CVI. However, the United States would still maintain an effective basic and applied vaccine research capability, which may produce technological spin-offs relevant to the CVI.

STRATEGY 2: FORGING NEW PARTNERSHIPS BETWEEN THE PUBLIC AND PRIVATE SECTORS

A significant obstacle to encouraging private-sector involvement in the development of CVI vaccines is that most of these products are currently of little commercial interest. Considerable resources are required to bring a candidate vaccine from the laboratory bench to the point at which it can be used to protect a child from disease. Given this level of investment and the relatively small profit margins associated with vaccines used predominately in the developing world, there are few incentives for the private sector to develop CVI vaccines.

Currently, U.S. strengths in vaccine-related activities lie in the public and private resources devoted to and available for research, development, and manufacture. Therefore, for the United States to contribute fully to the CVI, ways must be found to eliminate or reduce some of the costs and risks associated with vaccine development and pilot production. Realistically, only then would U.S. vaccine manufacturers consider assuming the scaleup of a final CVI vaccine product. Two options were identified: (1) establish a brokering mechanism, supported by incentives attractive to industry, to bring the private and public sectors together to develop CVI products, and (2) establish a facility to conduct CVI research and development and to produce pilot lots of vaccine. Such an entity could be independent, or it could be located within an existing government agency.

Both options hold the promise of facilitating the development of new vaccines against diseases of primary importance in developing countries as well as improvements in existing vaccines. Establishing partnerships between the public and private sectors through a brokering arrangement or establishing a CVI research and development facility would encourage the creation of technologically simple, low-cost vaccine technologies that could be easily transferred to vaccine manufacturers in developing countries. Either approach would permit the exploitation of vaccine technologies that are nonproprietary and therefore of little interest to commercial manufacturers who desire market exclusivity. Finally, either would allow the development of "orphan" vaccines that have very small or nonprofitable markets.

Option 1: Broker CVI R&D and Pilot Manufacture

A CVI division within any of a number of government organizations (AID, CDC, DOD, FDA, NIH, or the National Vaccine Program [NVP]) or as an independent entity, could administer a program of grants and contracts supporting applied research and development that would focus on two or three high-priority CVI vaccines. Such an entity might operate similarly to the Defense Advanced Research Projects Agency (see Box D-1).

Money would be awarded on a competitive basis to development-stage firms, pharmaceutical companies, university-based researchers, or government research laboratories. A peer-review system, similar to that used at NIH, could be used to evaluate the scientific merit of proposals. This CVI division could provide a market for new vaccines by guaranteeing the purchase of a given volume over a specified number of years and at a predetermined price. To be truly effective as a grants management entity for the CVI, the CVI division would offer incentives to the private sector (see box), retain patent rights for products resulting from CVI unit-funded research, and have the ability to license products to developing countries.

This option would strenthen and broaden an already solid U.S. research and development capability in vaccines. By guaranteeing a stable market for over a period of years and providing grants and various incentives, this option would both enable and encourage development-stage companies to develop CVI vaccines. One critical factor that this option does not address is the shortage of pilot production facilities in the United States. Those parties that are willing to take part in developing CVI vaccines, but that do not have in-house pilot production capabilities, would only be able to develop the products up to the point of pilot manufacture.

Both options in this strategy would require an infusion of public funds into the U.S. vaccine development system. This option would also require that a relevant government agency be willing and able to accommodate a CVI division.

Contribution to the Global CVI

This option would capitalize on the unique expertise and capabilities in the U.S. private sector and make maximal use of existing resources in the U.S. public sector in advancing CVI vaccine research and development. If these vaccines are indeed successfully developed, they would be accessible

---

Box D-1 Defense Advanced Research Projects Agency

The Defense Advanced Research Projects Agency (DARPA) was established in 1958 after the Soviet Union's launch of Sputnik. One of the primary motives for establishing DARPA was to develop technologies to serve missions in which no single uniformed service was interested or missions that spanned the needs of several services. Moreover, DARPA was primarily concerned with the "early-stage" development of new technologies; their incorporation into specific weapons systems was the responsibility of the uniformed services' research and technology facilities.

Today, DARPA functions a "technology-broker" or venture capitalist within the Pentagon, monitoring and funding the early development of high-risk, advanced technologies with applications to military systems. DARPA does not carry out research in its own facilities but contracts work to industry, universities, and branches of the armed services. DARPA has a full-time staff of 132 and manages an annual budget of $1.43 billion.

Overall, DARPA is an efficient organization that has minimized bureaucratic obstacles to program success. It has been able to attract talented scientists and engineers from outside government. An important reason for DARPA's success is that the Defense Department serves as a test customer for the technologies developed by DARPA. Projects benefit from feedback of user needs generated by a strong customer-client relationship.

Source: Reprinted with permission from *The Government Role in Civilian Technology: Building a New Alliance.* Copyright 1992 by the National Academy of Sciences. Courtesy of the National Academy Press, Washington, D.C.

---

to the developing world through licensing agreements.

Option 2: Develop an Entity with CVI-Related R&D and Pilot Manufacturing Capabilities

In the event that the grants and contracts mechanism fails to stimulate sufficient private-sector interest, the creation of a publicly funded entity to conduct R&D and pilot manufacture for subsequent handoff to commercial manufacturers may be necessary. Access to pilot production facilities would

Box D-2   Existing and Proposed Incentives to the Private Sector

Orphan Drug Act (1983)   Enacted in 1983 as Public Law 97-414, the Orphan Drug Act was designed to provide incentives to the pharmaceutical industry to develop drugs against diseases affecting fewer than 200,000 citizens in the United States.   Among the incentives offered are research grants, a 50 percent income-tax credit on most clinical research expenditures, assistance with FDA approval, and exclusive license to market the product for 7 years, which begins the moment the drug is approved by the FDA.   It is this 7-year exclusivity which has since emerged to be the most powerful incentive to industry.   According to the Pharmaceutical Manufacturer's Association, 64 orphan drugs have been developed and an additional 189 are under development (Pharmaceutical Manufacturers Association, 1992).   There is criticism, however, that many orphan drugs, developed with considerable assistance from the U.S. government, are not fiscal orphans at all.   A number of these products have been exceedingly profitable for their manufacturers.

Small Business Innovation Research Program   Enacted in 1982 as part of the Small Business Innovation Development Act (P.L. 97-219), the Small Business Innovation Research (SBIR) program seeks to encourage small businesses to engage in technological innovation and to commercialize discoveries originating in federally funded research and development through various mechanisms including grants, cooperative agreements, and contracts.   To be eligible for the SBIR program, businesses must have fewer than 500 employees, be 51 percent U.S. owned, and conduct all research and development in the United States. The U.S. government retains a royalty-free license on all patent rights resulting from SBIR-funded research for federal use and reserves the right to require the patent holder to license rights in certain circumstances.

Guaranteed Procurement   Under a procurement guarantee, the U.S. government could guarantee 5-year downstream purchasing of a given number of doses of a desired vaccine at a set price.   This could include a "cost-plus x" agreement, where "x" would be in the range of 12–15 percent of returns on investment.   However, cost-plus agreements generally do not offer incentives to manufacturers to hold costs down. Such a guarantee could also include provisions for licensing and transfer of the vaccine technology and the vaccine product to developing nations.

Patent Extension In response to taking up the challenge of developing and manufacturing a CVI vaccine at an affordable price, the government could extend a company's patent on an existing product (either a vaccine or a drug) for a set period of time. Such a patent extension would have to be negotiated early on and publicized so as to avoid charges of unfair competition from the generic drug industry.

Income-Tax Credits Establishment of a tax credit based on participation in the CVI could be a strong incentive to those companies that have a tax liability. Many smaller companies, however, in particular biotechnology companies have a relatively precarious financial position, and may be unable to take advantage of such a credit. These companies may be more receptive to investment tax credits.

overcome one of the major bottlenecks in the development of the low-profit vaccines that are usually sidelined in the few facilities that exist, giving way to more commercially viable products.

With its own vaccine research and development and pilot manufacturing capabilities, the entity would enable the public sector to share the risk of developing vaccines that have marginal profitability. The entity could draw on relevant expertise in government laboratories and agencies and the private sector, perhaps through visiting scientists. Nationals from developing countries would be trained in the facility by U.S. government and industry scientists. The entity would manufacture only those products for which a commercial partner has not been vigorously sought and identified.

The entity would have the ability to enter into cooperative research and development agreements, license technology, and retain revenues from vaccines sales or licensing. In addition, it would require the ability to hire qualified staff at competitive salaries, purchase needed equipment, make facility renovations, and build new facilities with minimal interference from bureaucratic procedures and timetables. Finally, the center would need a mechanism for protection from vaccine injury-related liability. There are successful precedents for such federally chartered institutions that operate with a significant amount of independence, including the Henry M. Jackson Foundation at the Uniformed Services University of the Health Sciences and the Tennessee Valley Authority (see boxes).

Because facilitating technology transfer of center-developed products and technologies would be one of the center's functions, perhaps matching grants could be solicited from bilateral and multilateral organizations such as the World Health Organization, the United Nations Children's Fund, the United Nations Development Program, and AID to assist in funding technology

---

Box D-3 Henry M. Jackson Foundation

Chartered by Congress to advance military medicine, the Henry M. Jackson Foundation was written into law on May 27, 1983. The foundation is modeled after the Smithsonian Institution, in that it is a federally chartered, nonprofit, nongovernmental organization authorized to receive federal or other funds; in return, it provides the government or other funders services on a contract basis. Typically, the foundation enters into cooperative ventures with the Uniformed Services University of the Health Sciences and other public or private entities to carry out projects in medical research, consultation or education. Flexibility is vital to the Foundation's strength, as it can employ both federal and nonfederal employees, receive patents, and negotiate licenses.   In addition, it is not constrained by personnel ceilings and has flexibility in salarly levels, and because it is a nonprofit foundation, its overhead rates are relatively low. There is continued congressional interest in the foundation's activities because the Chairmen and ranking minority members of the Senate and House Armed Services Committees serve on the foundation's Council of Directors.

---

transfer activities.

Among the potential concerns regarding the creation of a new entity are the requirements for funding and the view that it would only add to an already large number of organizations and institutions involved in vaccine-related activities in the United States.

Contribution to the Global CVI

A new center for CVI research and development and pilot manufacture could lend considerable support to the CVI Product Development Groups and developing-country vaccine manufacturers. Also, as in option 1, the technology would be transferred to the developing world, through both licensing agreements and visiting scientist programs.

STRATEGY 3: EMBARK ON A PUBLIC-SECTOR MODEL

Vaccines with a strong commercial market are developed in the United States by the private sector; those without such a market are not. Given

Box D-4 The Tennessee Valley Authority

The Tennessee Valley Authority (TVA) was established in 1933 as part of the U.S. government's attempt to lift the country out of the Great Depression. The TVA was to be a unique entity–"a corporation clothed with the power of government but possessed of the flexibility and initiative of a private enterprise." This new federal corporation was made an independent agency, reporting directly to the President and the U.S. Congress. Rather than several agencies trying to deal with the variety of public needs in the region, one unified development body would serve the whole area.

In 1959, Congress passed an amendment to the TVA Act that gave the TVA the power to issue its own bonds for money to construct its own power plants. Prior to the amendment, the TVA was forced to rely on congressional appropriations for new plants; the new legislation made the TVA power system "self-financing." In other words, the TVA could reach its own conclusions about when and where to build new facilities. It is important to note, however, that the amendment also defined the geographical boundaries of the TVA's power service area: there would be no more territorial expansion into areas served by private companies.

Through today, the TVA's mandate remains the management of the Tennessee River and working with state and local governments in resource development programs. Current TVA projects include (1) electric cars and experimental batteries being tested on TVA facilities; (2) researching strategies to convert wood and farm products into alcohol for fuel; and (3) the operation of a pilot plant to test methods for burning coal more efficiently, causing less pollution while generating electricity. In addition, the TVA runs one of the nation's main training centers for nuclear plant personnel.

Now a significant player in the electric utility industry, the TVA's electricity sale revenues were $5.1 billion on 112.4 billion kilowatt-hours, while its net income was $120 million in fiscal year 1992. Congress appropriated $135 million to the TVA for that same year, and as of September 1992, the TVA employed approximately 19,500 people.

Sources: TVA Annual Report, 1992; TVA Annual Report, 1953; A Student History of TVA, a TVA Information Office publication.

that the development and manufacture of new and improved vaccines are critical to the health and welfare of children in the United States and abroad, it could be argued that the public sector should assume responsibility for public health needs that are not met by the private sector. (The Public Health Service Act of 1944 permits the government to produce vaccines and other products not available from licensed establishments [See Appendix E].)

A public-sector agency could take on every stage of the vaccine life cycle: set priorities, generate requirements for vaccines, conduct basic and applied research, and engage in product development, full-scale manufacture of vaccines, and delivery. A public-sector vaccine developer and manufacturer would be responsive to the public health needs of the U.S. population as well as to those of the developing world.

Vaccines manufactured by the public sector could be sold on a cost-plus basis to public health departments in the developing world, international agencies, and/or commercial distributors in developing countries. To use the vaccines for this purpose without being hindered by the cost of having to obtain licenses, the public sector must have a mechanism to ensure ownership of intellectual property rights of all antigens and technologies contained in the vaccines.

Despite the potential attractiveness of a vaccine manufacturer that would respond to unmet public health needs, the public sector does not have the experience in the large-scale manufacture of vaccines. In addition, efficient vaccine production does not lend itself to government procurement policies and bureaucracy, and this strategy does little to capitalize on the research, development, and manufacturing capabilites that already exist in the private sector. Furthermore, it may be politically untenable to commit such substantial U.S. government resources to products with no demand in the United States. Most importantly, however, this model does not take advantage of the unique skills and capabilities in the private sector, including both biotechnology firms and commercial vaccine manufacturers.

Contribution to the Global CVI

The U.S. government would develop and manufacture CVI vaccines and sell them to UNICEF and developing countries at an affordable price.

* * *

Over the course of the study, the committee considered each of the major strategies and options outlined above–their contribution to the global CVI and the extent to which each takes maximal advantage of U.S. public and private sector expertise and resources. The committee's recommended strategy, which draws on elements of the strategies and options considered above, is discussed in greater detail in Chapter 7 of this report.

E

Public Health Service Act (1944)

PUBLIC LAWS–CH. 373–JULY 1, 1944
PART F–BIOLOGICAL PRODUCTS
Regulation of Biological Products

Sale, barter or
exchange in D.C., etc.

Sec. 351. (a) No person shall sell, barter, or offer for sale, barter, or exchange in the District of Columbia, or send, carry, or bring for sale, barter, or exchange from any State or possession into any other State or possession or into any foreign country, or from any foreign country into any State or possession, any virus, therapeutic serum, toxin, antitoxin, or analogous product, or arsphenamine or its derivatives (or any other trivalent organic arsenic compound), applicable to the prevention,

Manufacturers of
virus, etc.
License require-
ments.

treatment, or cure of diseases or injuries of man, unless (1) such virus, serum, toxin, antitoxin, or other product has been propagated or manufactured and prepared at an establishment holding an unsuspended and unrevoked license, issued by the Administrator as hereinafter authorized, to propogate or manufacture, and prepare such virus, serum, toxin, antitoxin, or other product for sale in the District of Columbia, or for sending, bringing

Package marking requirement.

or carrying from place to place aforesaid; and (2) each package of such virus, serum, toxin, antitoxin, or other product is plainly marked with the proper name of the article contained therein, the name, address, and license number of the manufacturer, and the date beyond which the specific results. The

Effect of license suspension, etc.

suspension or revocation of any license shall not prevent the sale, barter, or exchange of any virus, serum, toxin, antitoxin, or other product aforesaid which has been sold and delivered by the licensee prior to such suspension or revocation, unless the owner or custodian of such virus, serum, toxin, antitoxin, or other product aforesaid has been notified by the Administrator not to sell, barter, or exchange the same.

False labels, etc.

(b) No person shall falsely label or mark any package or container of any virus, serum, toxin, antitoxin, or other product aforesaid; nor alter any label or mark on any package or container or any virus, serum, toxin, antitoxin, or other product aforesaid so as to falsify such label or mark.

Inspection of establishments for manufacture of virus, etc.

(c) Any officer, agent, or employee or the Federal Security Agency, authorized by the Administrator for the purpose, may during all reasonable hours enter and inspect any establishment for the propagation or manufacture and preparation of any virus, serum, toxin, antitoxin, or other product aforesaid for sale, barter, or exchange in the District of Columbia, or to be sent, carried, or brought from any State or possession into any other State or possession or into any foreign country, or from any foreign country into any State or possession.

Issuance of licenses, standards required.

(d) Licenses for the maintenance of establishments for the propagation or manufacture and preparation of products described in subsection (a) of this section may be issued only upon a showing desired meet standards, designed to insure the continued safety, purity, and potency of such products, prescribed in regulations made jointly by the Surgeon General, the Surgeon General of the Army, and the Surgeon General of the Navy, and approved by the Administrator, and licenses for new products may be issued only upon a showing that they meet such standards. All such licenses shall be issued, suspended, and revoked as prescribed by regulations and all licenses issued for the maintenance of establishments for the propagation or manufacture and preparation, in any foreign country, or any such produccts for sale, barter, or exchange in any State or possession shall be issued upon condition that the licensees will permit the inspection of their establishments in accordance with subsection (c) of this section.

Interference With Officers

(e) No person shall interfere with any officer, agent, or employee of the Service in the performance of any duty imposed upon him by this section or by regulations made by authority thereof.

Penalties for Offenses

(f) Any person who shall violate, or aid or abet in violating, any of the provisions of this section shall be punished upon conviction by a fine not exceeding $500 or by imprisonment not exceeding one year, or by both such fine and imprisonment, in the discretion of the court.

(g) Nothing contained in this Act shall be construed as in any way affecting, modifying, repealing, or superseding the provisions of the Federal Food, Drug and Cosmetic Act (U.S.C., 1940 edition, title 21, ch. 9).

(h)(1)(A)[1] A partially processed biological product which is not in a form applicable to the prevention, treatment, or cure of diseases or injuries of man, which is not intended for sale in the United States, and which is intended for further manufacture into final dosage form outside the United States in a country listed under section

---

[1] Added by sec. 105 of P.L. 99-660.

802(b)(A) of the Federal Food, Drug, and Cosmetic Act may, upon approval of an application meeting the requirements of subparagraph (B), be exported to a country listed under section 802(b)(4) of the Federal Food, Drug, and Cosmetic Act. The Secretary may not approve an application to export such a product unless the Secretary determines that the product is manufactured, processed, packaged, and held in conformity with current good manufacturing practice and the outside of the shipping package is labeled with the following statement: "This product may be sold or offered for sale only in the following countries: ," the blank space being filled with a list of the countries to which export of the drug is authorized.

(B) An application for the export of a partially processed biological product shall–

(i) describe the partially processed biological product to be exported,

(ii) list each country to which the product is to be exported,

(iii) contain a certification by the applicant that the product will not be exported to a country not listed under clause (ii),

(iv) identify the establishments in which the product is manufactured, and

(v) contain a certification by the applicant that the final product to be developed from the partially processed product is approved in the country to which it is to be exported or approval of the final product is being sought in such country.

(2) A product described in paragraph (1) is not subject to licensure under this section.

(3) If the Secretary determines that prohibiting the export of a product described in paragraph (1) is necessary for protection of the public health in the United States or the country to which it is to be exported, the Secretary may not approve an application under paragraph (1) for the export of

such product.

Preparation of Biological Products by Service

Sec. 352. [263] (a) The Service may prepare for its own use any product described in section 351 and any product necessary to carrying out any of the purposes of section 301.

(b) The Service may prepare any product described in section 351 for the use of other Federal departments or agencies, and public or private agencies and individuals engaged in work in the field of medicine when such product is not available from establishments licensed under such section.

F

National Vaccine Program Legislation

Establishment

Sec. 2101. [300aa-1] The Secretary shall establish in the Department of Health and Human Services a National Vaccine Program to achieve optimal prevention of human infectious diseases through immunization and to achieve optimal prevention against adverse reactions to vaccines. The Program shall be administered by a Director selected by the Secretary.

Program Responsibilities

Sec. 2102. [300aa-2] (a) The Director of the Program shall have the following responsibilities:

(1) Vaccine Research. –The Director of the Program shall, through the plan issued under section 2103, coordinate and provide directon for research carried out in or through the National Institutes of Health, the Centers for Disease Control, the Office of Biologics Research and Review of the Food and Drug Administration, the Department of Defense, and the Agency for International Development on means to induce human immunity against

naturally occurring infectious diseases and to prevent adverse reactions to vaccines.

(2) Vaccine Development. –The Director of the Program shall, through the plan issued under section 2103, coordinate and provide direction for activities carried out in or through the National Institutes of Health, the Office of Biologics Research and Review of the Food and Drug Administration, the Department of Defense, and the Agency for International Development to develop the techniques needed to produce safe effective vaccines.

(3) Safety and Efficacy Testing of Vaccines. –The Director of the Program shall, through the plan issued under section 2103, coordinate and provide direction for safety and efficacy testing of vaccines carried out in or through the National Institutes of Health, the Centers for Disease Control, the Office of Biologics Research and Review of the Food and Drug Administration, the Department of Defense, and the Agency for International Development.

(4) Licensing of Vaccine Manufacturers and Vaccines. –The Director of the Program shall, through the plan issued under section 2103, coordinate and provide direction for the allocation of resources in the implementation of the licensing program under section 353.

(5) Production and Procurement of Vaccines. –The Director of the Program shall, through the plan issued under section 2103 ensure that the governmental and non-governmental production and procurement of safe and effective vaccines by the Public Health Service, the Department of Defense, and the Agency for International Development meet the needs of the United States population and fulfill commitments of the United States to prevent human infectious diseases in other countries.

(6) Distribution and Use of Vaccines. –The Director of the Program shall, through the plan issued under section 2103, coordinate and provide direction to the Centers for Disease Control and assistance to States, localities, and health practitioners in the distribution and use of vaccines, including efforts to encourage public acceptance of immunizations and to make health practitioners and the public aware of potential adverse reactions and contraindications to vaccines.

(7) Evaluation of the Need for and the Effectiveness and Adverse Effects of Vaccines and Immunization Activities. –The Director of the Program shall, through the plan issued under section 2103, coordinate and provide direction to the National Institutes of Health, the Centers for Disease Control, the Office of Biologics Research and Review of the Food and Drug Administration, the National Center for Health Statistics, the National Center for Health Services Research and Health Care Technology Assessment, and the Health Care Financing Administration in monitoring the need for and the effectiveness and adverse effects of vaccines and

immunization activities.

(8) Coordinating Governmental and Non-Governmental Activities. –The Director of the Program shall, through the plan issued under section 2103, provide for the exchange of information between Federal agencies involved in the implementation of the Program and non-governmental entities engaged in the development and production of vaccines and in vaccine research and encourage the investment of non-governmental resources complementary to the governmental activities under the Program.

(9) Funding of Federal Agencies. –The Director of the Program shall make available to Federal agencies involved in the implementation of the plan issued under section 2103 funds appropriated under section 2106 to supplement the funds otherwise available to such agencies for activities under the plan.

(b) In carrying out subsection (a) and in preparing the plan under section 2103, the Director shall consult with all Federal agencies involved in research on and development, testing licensing, production, procurement, distribution, and use of vaccines.

Plan

Sec. 2103. [300aa-3] The Director of the Program shall prepare and issue a plan for the implementation of the responsibilities of the Director under section 2102. The plan shall establish priorities in research and the development, testing, licensing, production, procurement, distribution, and effective use of vaccines, describe an optimal use of resources to carry out such priorities, and describe how each of the various departments and agencies will carry out their vaccine functions in consultation and coordination with the Program and in conformity with such priorities. The first plan under this section shall be prepared not later than January 1, 1987, and shall be revised not later than January 1 of each succeeding year.

Report

Sec. 2104. [300aa-4] The Director shall report to the Committee on Energy and Commerce of the House of Representatives and the Committee on Labor and Human Resources of the Senate not later than January 1, 1988, and annually thereafter on the implementation of the Program and the plan prepared under section 2103.

National Vaccine Advisory Committee

Sec. 2105. [300aa-5] There is established the National Vaccine Advisory Committee. The members of the Committee shall be appointed by the Director of the Program, in consultation with the National Academy of Sciences, from among individuals who are engaged in vaccine research or the manufacture of vaccines or who are physicians, members of parent organizations concerned with immunizations, or representatives of State or local health agencies or public health organizations.

(b) The Committee shall—

(1) study and recommend ways to encourage the availability of an adequate supply of safe and effective vaccination products in the States,

(2) recommend research priorities and other measures the Director of the Program should take to enhance safety and efficacy of vaccines,

(3) advise the Director of the Program in the implementation of sections 2102, 2103, and 2104, and

(4) identify annually for the Director of the Program the most important areas of government and non-government cooperation that should be considered in implementing sections 2102, 2103, and 2104.

Authorizations

Sec. 2106. [300aa-6] (a) To carry out this subtitle other than section 2102(9) there are authorized to be appropriated $4,000,000 for fiscal year 1991, and such sums as may be necessary for each of the fiscal years 1992 through 1995.

(b) To carry out section 2102(9) there are authorized to be appropriated $30,000,000 for fiscal year 1991, and such sums as may be necessary for each of the fiscal years 1992 through 1995.

G

Immunization Schedules

Table G-1 provides the immunization schedule recommended by the Advisory Committee on Immunization Practices (ACIP). Table G-2 provides the immunization recommendations of the American Academy of Pediatrics (AAP). Also provided in this Appendix is the immunization schedule recommended by the Pan American Health Organization and the the World Health Organization.

TABLE G-1   Immunization Schedule Recommended by ACIP

Age	Vaccine
Birth	HBV
2 months	HBV, DTP, OPV, HibCV
4 months	HBV, DTP, OPV, HibCV
6 months	HBV, DTP, HibCV
12 months	HibCV
15 months	DTaP or DTP, OPV, MMR, HibCV
4–6 years	DTaP or DTP, OPV, MMR
14–16 years (every 10 years throughout life)	Td

NOTE: The recommended ages are not absolute; for example, age 2 months can be ages 6–10 weeks. All recommended vaccines can be given simultaneously. Hepatitis B vaccine may be given in either of 2 schedules: birth, 1-2 months, 6–18 months or 1-2 months, 4 months, 6–18 months. HibOC is given at 2,4,6, and 15 months; PRP-OMP is given at 2,4, and 12 months. DTaP is recommended for 15 months and 4–6 years, but whole-cell DTP may still be used if DTaP is not available.

SOURCE: Adapted from the ACIP Recommended Immunization Schedule. Copies can be obtained from: National Immunization Program, Centers for Disease Control and Prevention, Mailstop E-05, 1600 Clifton Road, Atlanta, GA 30333.

TABLE G-2 Immunization Schedule Recommended by AAP

Age	DTP	Polio	MMR	Hepatitis B[a]	Haemophilus	Tetanus-Diphtheria
Birth				X		
1–2 months				X		
2 months	X	X			X	
4 months	X	X			X	
6 months	X				X[b]	
6–18 months				X		
12–15 months					X[b]	
15 months			X		X[b]	
15–18 months	X[c]	X				
4–6 years	X[c]	X				
11–12 years			X[d]			
14–16 years						X

[a] Infants of mothers who tested seropositive for hepatitis B (HBsAg+) must receive hepatitis B immune globulin (HBIG) at or shortly after the first dose. These infants also will require a second hepatitis B vaccine dose at 1 month and a third hepatitis B vaccine injection at 6 months of age.

[b] Depends on previous *Haemophilus influenzae* type b vaccine given.

[c] For the fourth and fifth dose, the acellular (DTaP) pertussis vaccine may be substituted for the DTP vaccine.

[d] Except where public health authorities require otherwise.

SOURCE: Used with permission of the American Academy of Pediatrics. Schedule.

TABLE G-3 Immunization Schedule Recommended for EPI

Contact	Age	Vaccines
1	Birth	BCG and OPV
2	6 weeks	DTP and OPV
3	10 weeks	DTP and OPV
4	14 weeks	DTP and OPV
5	9 months	Measles

SOURCE: Expanded Program on Immunization, World Health Organization; Pan American Health Organization. Provided by Ciro de Quadros, Pan American Health Organization.

H

Historical Record of Vaccine Product License Holders in the United States

TABLE H-1 Vaccine Product License Holders in the United States

Company and Vaccine or Product	Date of License	Date of Revocation
Bionetics Research Inc.[a]		
BCG vaccine	05/29/1987	06/21/1989
Connaught Laboratories, Inc.[b]		
BCG live	05/21/1990	
BCG vaccine	03/31/1967	05/21/1990
Diphtheria & tetanus toxoids & acellular pertussis vaccine, adsorbed	09/20/1992	
Diphtheria & tetanus toxoids & pertussis vaccine (DTP)	01/03/1978	11/29/1982
Diphtheria & tetanus toxoids, & pertussis vaccine, adsorbed	01/03/1978	
Diphtheria & tetanus toxoids adsorbed	09/18/1984	
Diphtheria toxoid	01/03/1978	
Haemophilus influenzae type b Conjugate (diphtheria toxoid conjugate)	12/22/1987	

TABLE H-1 *Continued*

Company and Vaccine or Product	Date of License	Date of Revocation
Haemophilus influenzae		
type b polysaccharide	12/20/1985	
Influenza	01/03/1978	
Meningococcal polysaccharide group A	01/03/1978	
Meningococcal polysaccharide group C	01/03/1978	
Meningococcal polysaccharide vaccine,		
groups A and C combined	01/03/1978	
Meningococcal polysaccharide vaccine, groups		
A, C, Y, W135 combined	11/23/1981	
Pertussis vaccine	01/03/1978	
Poliomyelitis virus, inactivated		
human diploid cell	11/20/1987	
Poliomyelitis virus, inactivated		
monkey kidney cell	01/24/1963	
Rabies vaccine	12/27/1991	
Smallpox vaccine	01/03/1978	
Tetanus toxoid	01/03/1978	
Tetanus toxoid, adsorbed	01/03/1978	
Tetanus & diphtheria toxoids adsorbed		
(for adult use)	01/03/1978	
Yellow fever	01/03/1978	
Connaught Laboratories, Limited[b]		
Diphtheria toxoid	04/28/1928	05/27/1977
Tetanus toxoid	01/14/1943	
Small pox vaccine	10/23/1967	04/01/1980
Dow Chemical Company[a]		
Diphtheria & tetanus toxoids &		
pertussis vaccine adsorbed	09/11/1970	06/07/1977
Diphtheria toxoid	09/18/1934	06/07/1977
DT, adsorbed	09/11/1970	06/07/1977
DP, adsorbed	09/11/1970	06/07/1977
Measles, live	02/05/1965	06/07/1978
Measles and rubella, live	04/17/1974	06/21/1978
Measles, mumps, rubella, live	04/17/1974	06/21/1978
Mumps virus vaccine, live	04/17/1974	06/21/1978
Pertussis vaccine	10/01/1932	06/07/1977
Rubella virus, live	03/01/1974	06/21/1978
Tetanus toxoid	08/01/1936	06/07/1977
Tetanus toxoid, adsorbed	09/01/1970	06/07/1977
Eli Lilly and Company[a]		
Cholera	10/31/1917	06/07/1979
Diphtheria & tetanus toxoids	09/09/1970	06/07/1979

Continues

TABLE H-1 *Continued*

Company and Vaccine or Product	Date of License	Date of Revocation
Diphtheria & tetanus toxoids and pertussis vaccine adsorbed	09/09/1970	12/02/1985
DT, adsorbed	09/09/1970	06/07/1979
Influenza	11/09/1945	04/11/1977
Mumps vaccine	01/27/1950	04/11/1977
Pertussis vaccine	03/31/1915	03/07/1978
Rabies vaccine	06/07/1915	08/11/1982
Streptococcus vaccine	04/17/1952	10/27/1988
Tetanus toxoid	12/10/1935	06/07/1979
Tetanus toxoid, adsorbed	09/09/1970	06/07/1979
Tetanus & diphtheria toxoid adsorbed (for adult use)	09/09/1970	06/07/1979
Typhoid	02/04/1954	11/13/1978
Typhus	03/11/1941	06/07/1979
Evans Medical Ltd.[c]		
Influenza	08/12/1988	
Glaxo Operations, U.K. Ltd.[a]		
BCG vaccine	01/24/1963	07/17/1990
Lederle Laboratories,[d]		
American Cyanamid Company		
Cholera	12/26/1941	
Diphtheria & tetanus toxoids and acellular pertussis, adsorbed	12/17/1991	
Diphtheria & tetanus toxoids and pertussis vaccine adsorbed	07/24/1970	
DT, adsorbed	07/29/1970	
Haemophilus influenzae type b polysaccharide vaccine	12/20/1985	
Influenza	12/07/1945	
Measles virus, live	05/03/1966	05/21/1980
Mumps vaccine	06/22/1950	05/24/1978
Pertussis vaccine	01/19/1914	05/29/1980
Pneumococcal vaccine, polyvalent	08/15/1979	
Polio virus, live, oral trivalent	06/25/1963	
Polio virus, oral, type 1	03/27/1962	
Polio virus, oral, type 2	03/27/1962	
Polio virus, oral, type 3	03/27/1962	
Rocky mountain spotted fever	04/13/1942	06/11/1979
Small pox	03/01/1937	05/24/1978
Tetanus toxoid	06/15/1935	
Tetanus toxoid, adsorbed	07/29/1970	

TABLE H-1 *Continued*

Company and Vaccine or Product	Date of License	Date of Revocation
Tetanus & Diphtheria toxoids adsorbed		
(for adult use)	07/29/1970	
Typhus	05/24/1967	11/20/1980
Massachusetts Public Health Biologic Laboratories		
Diphtheria & tetanus toxoids		
& pertussis vaccine adsorbed	07/27/1970	
Diphtheria toxoid	07/07/1932	05/19/1980
DT, adsorbed	07/27/1970	
Small pox	03/20/1917	12/22/1976
Tetanus toxoid	05/16/1949	10/11/1989
Tetanus toxoid, adsorbed	07/29/1970	
Tetanus & diphtheria toxoids adsorbed		
(for adult use)	07/27/1970	
Typhoid	03/20/1917	10/26/1988
Merck and Company		
Cholera	05/04/1952	01/31/1986
Diphtheria & tetanus toxoids		
and pertussis vaccine adsorbed	08/31/1970	01/31/1986
Haemophilus influenzae type b		
conjugate (meningococcal		
protein conjugate)	12/20/1989	
Hepatitis B vaccine	11/16/1981	
Hepatitis B recombinant	07/23/1986	
Influenza	11/30/1945	
Measles, live and small pox	11/17/1967	03/12/1987
Measles virus, live	03/21/1963	
Measles and mumps virus, live	07/18/1973	
Measles and rubella virus, live	04/22/1971	
Measles, mumps, rubella, live	04/22/1971	
Meningococcal polysaccharide A	07/11/1975	
Meningococcal polysaccharide C	04/02/1974	
Meningococcal polysaccharide A&C	10/06/1975	
Meningococcal polycsaccharide		
A, C, Y, W135 combined	12/14/1982	
Mumps virus, live	12/28/1967	
Pneumococcal	11/21/1977	
Poliomyelitis, inactivated		
monkey kidney cell	04/12/1955	07/29/1980
Rubella virus, live	06/09/1969	
Rubella and mumps, live	08/30/1970	
Small pox	09/21/1965	07/29/1980
Tetanus toxoid	12/11/1933	01/31/1986
Tetanus toxoid, adsorbed	08/31/1970	01/31/1986

Continues

TABLE H-1 *Continued*

Company and Vaccine or Product	Date of License	Date of Revocation
Tetanus & diphtheria toxoids adsorbed		
(for adult use)	08/31/1970	01/31/1986
Typhoid	04/25/1963	01/31/1986
Typhus	12/24/1941	07/29/1980
Merrell National Laboratories,		
Division of Richardson Merrell[a]		
Cholera	02/27/1942	03/25/1976
DTP	10/15/1970	01/03/1978
Diphtheria & tetanus toxoids & pertussis	05/16/1949	01/03/1978
vaccine adsorbed		
Diphtheria toxoid	09/28/1929	01/03/1978
Influenza	09/16/1947	01/03/1978
Meningococcal polysaccharide group A	09/19/1975	01/03/1978
Meningococcal polysaccharide group C	07/11/1975	01/03/1978
Meningococcal polysaccharide vaccine, groups		
A and C, combined	09/13/1976	01/03/1978
Pertussis vaccine	11/16/1926	01/03/1978
Small pox	03/05/1937	01/03/1978
Tetanus toxoid	05/25/1934	01/03/1978
Tetanus toxoid, adsorbed	10/15/1970	01/03/1978
Tetanus and diphtheria toxoids adsorbed		
(for adult use)	03/07/1955	01/03/1978
Yellow fever	05/22/1953	01/03/1978
Michigan Department of Public Health		
Anthrax	11/04/1970	
Diphtheria & tetanus toxoids		
and pertussis vaccine adsorbed	08/27/1970	
DT, adsorbed	08/27/1970	
Pertussis vaccine	11/22/1935	02/03/1977
Pertussis vaccine, adsorbed	10/12/1967	
Rabies vaccine, adsorbed	03/18/1988	
Smallpox	03/03/1937	06/25/1985
Tetanus toxoid, adsorbed	08/27/1970	
Typhoid	07/26/1926	06/25/1985
Miles Inc.[e]		
Cholera	10/03/1968	10/30/1970
Diphtheria and tetanus toxoids	06/01/1951	10/30/1970
DTP	05/04/1949	10/30/1970
Diphtheria & tetanus toxoids	05/04/1949	10/30/1970
and pertussis vaccine adsorbed		
Diphtheria toxoid	02/01/1928	10/30/1970
DT, adsorbed	05/04/1949	10/30/1970
DP, adsorbed	05/04/1949	10/30/1970

TABLE H-1 *Continued*

Company and Vaccine or Product	Date of License	Date of Revocation
Pertussis vaccine	08/03/1914	10/30/1970
Pertussis vaccine, adsorbed	05/03/1948	10/30/1970
Plague	05/14/1942	
Poliomyelitis, inactivated		
monkey kidney cell	04/12/1955	12/28/1978
Small pox	08/21/1903	06/11/1973
Tetanus toxoid	09/25/1940	11/01/1979
Tetanus toxoid, adsorbed	05/04/1949	10/30/1970
Tetanus & diphtheria toxoids adsorbed		
(for adult use)	11/16/1956	10/30/1970
Typhoid	03/06/1916	10/30/1970
Organon Teknika Corporation[e]		
BCG vaccine	06/21/1989	
Parke Davis, Division		
of Warner Lambert Company[a]		
Adenovirus	09/23/1957	07/29/1980
Adenovirus and influenza, combined		
aluminun phosphate adsorbed	09/22/1959	07/29/1980
Diphtheria and tetanus toxoids	07/29/1952	10/14/1981
DTP	07/29/1952	10/14/1981
Diphtheria & tetanus toxoids & pertussis	07/08/1952	10/14/1981
vaccine adsorbed		
Diphtheria toxoid	08/17/1927	10/14/1981
DT, adsorbed	07/08/1952	10/14/1981
DTP adsorbed, poliomyelitis	12/20/1963	10/14/1981
DTP, poliomyelitis adsorbed	03/25/1959	10/14/1981
Influenza	11/26/1945	
Pertussis	04/16/1952	10/14/1981
Pertussis vaccine, adsorbed	02/20/1952	10/14/1981
Poliomyelitis, adsorbed	10/04/1960	07/29/1980
Poliomyelitis, inactivated		
monkey kidney cell	04/12/1955	07/29/1980
Rabies vaccine	08/05/1942	03/21/1973
Tetanus toxoid	05/04/1940	10/14/1981
Tetanus toxoid, adsorbed	07/08/1952	10/14/1981
Typhoid	03/24/1916	02/24/1959
Typhus	03/25/1942	08/05/1947
Pasteur Merieux Vaccins et Serums, S.A.[b]		
Poliomyelitis, inactivated		
monkey kidney cell	12/21/1990	
Rabies vaccine	06/09/1980	

Continues

TABLE H-1 *Continued*

Company and Vaccine or Product	Date of License	Date of Revocation
Pfizer Ltd.[a]		
Poliovirus, live, oral trivalent	10/28/1966	06/12/1979
Poliovirus, oral type 1	08/17/1961	06/12/1979
Poliovirus, oral type 2	10/06/1961	06/12/1979
Poliovirus, oral type 3	03/27/1962	06/12/1979
Praxis Biologics, Incorporated[d]		
Haemophilus b conjugate vaccine		
(diphtheria CRM197 protein conjugate)	12/21/1988	
Haemophilus b polysaccharide vaccine	04/12/1985	
Research Foundation for Microbial Diseases, Osaka University		
Acellular pertussis vaccine concentrate	08/20/1992	
Japanese encephalitis virus vaccine inactivated	12/10/1992	
SCLAVO s.p.a[f]		
Cholera	08/19/1976	
Diphtheria and tetanus toxoids and		
pertussis vaccine adsorbed	03/31/1978	
Diphtheria toxoid	01/04/1963	
DT, adsorbed	03/31/1978	
Tetanus toxoid	01/04/1963	
Tetanus toxoid, adsorbed	08/05/1970	
Tetanus & diphtheria toxoids adsorbed		
(for adult use)	02/16/1979	
SmithKline Beecham[e]		
Hepatitis B, recombinant	08/28/1989	
Rubella virus, live	03/12/1970	10/05/1982
Swiss Serum Institute		
Tetanus toxoid, adsorbed	12/11/1970	
Typhoid vaccine, oral, Ty21a	12/15/1989	
Takeda Chemical Industries, Ltd., Acellular pertussis vaccine concentrate		
(for further manufacturing)	12/17/1991	
Texas Department of Health Resources		
Diphtheria & tetanus toxoids		
& pertussis vaccine adsorbed	07/27/1970	02/06/1979
Diphtheria toxoid	01/06/1963	02/06/1979
DT, adsorbed	07/27/1970	02/06/1979
Pertussis	12/27/1954	02/06/1979

TABLE H-1 *Continued*

Company and Vaccine or Product	Date of License	Date of Revocation
Tetanus toxoid	09/22/1959	02/06/1979
Tetanus & diphtheria toxoids adsorbed		
(for adult use)	07/27/1970	02/06/1979
Typhoid	07/11/1950	02/06/1979
University of Illinois[a]		
BCG vaccine	07/07/1950	05/29/1987
Wellcome[d]		
Rubella virus, live	03/01/1977	
Wyeth Laboratories		
Adenovirus, live, oral, type 4	07/01/1980	
Adenovirus, live, oral, type 7	07/01/1980	
Cholera	07/16/1952	
Diphtheria & tetanus toxoids		
and pertussis vaccine adsorbed	09/11/1970	
Diphtheria toxoid	05/19/1944	05/19/1987
DT, adsorbed	09/11/1970	
Influenza	12/13/1961	
Pertussis vaccine	07/16/1952	05/19/1987
Rabies vaccine	08/11/1982	08/07/1986
Smallpox	05/19/1944	
Tetanus toxoid	05/19/1944	
Tetanus toxoid, adsorbed	09/11/1970	
Tetanus & diphtheria toxoids adsorbed		
(for adult use)	09/11/1970	
Typhoid	07/16/1952	

[a] Company no longer produces any vaccines.
[b] Connaught Laboratories, Inc., (U.S.) and Connaught Laboratories, Ltd (Canada), are subsidiaries of Pasteur-Mérieux Sérums et Vaccins (France).
[c] Evans-Medical is a division of Medeva International, plc (United Kingdom); Medeva International plc acquired the vaccine business from Wellcome in 1991.
[d] Lederle Laboratories acquired Praxis Biologics in 1989. Lederle-Praxis Biologicals is now a business unit of American Cyanamid.
[e] Company produces one vaccine only for U.S. market.
[f] Sclavo spa is now owned by Ciba-Geigy (Switzerland) and Chiron (U.S.).

SOURCE: Center for Biologics Evaluation and Research, U.S. Food and Drug Administration, Bethesda, Maryland.

I

Working Group Participants
June 11–13, 1992

Claire Broome, M.D.
Associate Director for Science
Centers for Disease Control and
  Prevention
Atlanta, GA

Douglas L. Cocks, Ph.D.
Manager, Corporate Affairs
Eli Lilly
Indianapolis, IN

Ronald Ellis, Ph.D.
Executive Director
Virus and Cell Biology
Merck & Co., Inc.
West Point, PA

Peter Evans
World Health Organization
Geneva, Switzerland

Bernard Fritzell, Ph.D.
Director of Clinical Research
Connaught Laboratories, Inc.
Swiftwater, PA

Lance Gordon, Ph.D.
President and CEO
ORAVAX
Cambridge, MA

Carolyn Hardegree, M.D.
Director, Office of Biologics
  Research
U.S. Food & Drug
  Administration
Bethesda, MD

Akira Homma, M.D.
Regional Advisor in Biologics
Pan American Health
  Organization
Washington, DC

Pamela Johnson, Ph.D.
Chief, Applied Research Division
Office of Health
U.S. Agency for International
  Development
Washington, D.C.

Thomas D. Kiley, J.D.
Attorney
Hillsborough, CA

Pierre Lemoine
Chief, National Laboratory
  for Control of Vaccines
Ministry of Public Health
Brussels, Belgium

David Lohr
Vice President, Business
  Development
Medisorb Technologies
  International, Ltd.
Cincinnati, OH

Richard Mahoney, Ph.D.
Vice President and Director
Technology Promotion
Program for Appropriate
  Technology in Health
Seattle, WA

Harry M. Meyer, Jr., M.D.
President, Medical Research
  Division
American Cyanamid Co.
Pearl River, NY

David Mowery, Ph.D.
Associate Professor
University of California
  School of Business
Berkeley, CA

William Packer, C.P.A.
President
Virus Research Institute
Cambridge, MA

Timothy D. Proctor, J.D.
Associate General Counsel
Merck & Co., Inc.
Rahway, NJ

Philip K. Russell, M.D.
Professor, Division of
  International Health
John Hopkins School of Hygiene
  and Public Health
Baltimore, MD

Jerald C. Sadoff, M.D.
Director
Division of Communicable
  Diseases and Immunology
Walter Reed Army Institute
  for Research
Washington, DC

Jay P. Sanford, M.D.
Dean Emeritus
Uniformed Services University
  of the Health Sciences
Dallas, TX

Donald Shepard, Ph.D.
Professor
Institute for Health Policy
Brandeis University
Waltham, MA

Dale Spriggs, Ph.D.[1]
National Institute of Allergy and
  Infectious Diseases
Bethesda, Maryland

Ann Wion, J.D.
Associate Chief Counsel for
  Drugs and Biologics
U.S. Food & Drug
  Administration
Bethesda, MD

WORKING GROUP PARTICIPANTS
June 21–23, 1992

Frank Cano, Ph.D.[2]
Vice-President
Lederle-Praxis Biologicals
Pearl River, NY

Mary Lou Clements, M.D.
Professor and Head
Division of Vaccine Sciences
Johns Hopkins School of Hygiene
  and Public Health
Baltimore, MD

George Curlin, M.D.
Deputy Director
Division of Microbiology and
  Infectious Diseases
National Institute for Allergy
  and Infectious Diseases
Bethesda, MD

Ciro de Quadros, M.D.
Regional Advisor
Expanded Program on
  Immunization
Pan American Health
  Organization
Washington, DC

Michael Epstein, J.D.
Partner

Weil, Gotshal & Manges
New York, NY

Elaine Esber, M.D.
Associate Director
Center for Biologics Evaluation
  and Research
U.S. Food & Drug
  Administration
Bethesda, MD

Ronald W. Hansen, Ph.D.
Associate Dean for
  Academic Affairs
William E. Simon Graduate
  School of Business
University of Rochester
Rochester, NY

Kerri-Ann Jones, Ph.D.
Chief, Human Resources
Development, Energy and Private
  Sector
U.S. Agency for International
  Development
Washington, DC

David T. Karzon, M.D.
Professor
Vanderbilt University

School of Medicine
Nashville, TN

Scott Koenig
MedImmune, Inc.
Gaithersburg, MD

David S. Krause, M.D.
Director, Clinical Research,
  Development and Medical
  Affairs
SmithKline Beecham
King of Prussia, PA

Wendy K. Mariner, J.D.
Professor of Health Law
Boston University
School of Public Health
Boston, MA

Douglas Reynolds
Vice President of Marketing
Connaught Laboratories, Inc.
Swiftwater, PA

Bryan Roberts, Ph.D.
Research Director
Virus Research Institute
Cambridge, MA

Amy Scott
Consumer Safety Officer
U.S. Food & Drug
  Administration
Bethesda, MD

Jane Scott, Ph.D.
Senior Director, Vaccine
  Development
Lederle-Praxis Biologicals
Pearl River, NY

Seung-il Shin, Ph.D.[3]
Eugene Technologies
  International, Inc.,
Ramsey, NJ

George Siber, M.D.
Director, Biologic Laboratories
Massachusetts Department of
  Public Health
Jamaica Plain, MA

Jane E. Sisk, Ph.D.
Professor
Columbia University
  School of Public Health
New York, NY

Thomas Stagnaro
President and CEO
UNIVAX Biologics
Rockville, MD

Richard I. Walker, Ph.D.
Science Advisor
National Vaccine Program
National Institutes of Health
Rockville, MD

Michael White, M.D.
Medical Officer
Applied Research Division
Office of Health
U.S. Agency for International
  Development
Washington, D.C.

Douglas Williams
Vice President, Marketing
Connaught Laboratories, Inc.
Swiftwater, PA

James F. Young, Ph.D.
Vice President, Research &
  Development
MedImmune, Inc.
Gaithersburg, MD

NOTES

1. Dr. Spriggs is now with Virus Research Institute in Cambridge, MA.
2. Dr. Cano is now President, Aviron, Belmont, Ca.
3. Dr. Shin is now with the United Nations Development Program, New York, NY.

J

Committee and Staff Biographies

Mary Lou Clements, M.D., D.T.M.H., M.P.H., is Professor and Head of the Division of Vaccine Sciences, Department of International Health, and Director of the Center for Immunization Research at Johns Hopkins University School of Hygiene and Public Health. She received her M.D. from the University of Texas Southwestern Medical School, her D.T.M.H from the London School of Tropical Medicine and Hygiene, and her M.P.H. from Johns Hopkins University. She completed her medical training in internal medicine at Temple University Hospital in Philadelphia. From 1975 to 1977, she served as special epidemiologist for the World Health Organization's (WHO) Smallpox Eradication Program in India. Beginning in 1979, Dr. Clements was a faculty member at the University of Maryland School of Medicine at the Center for Vaccine Development; in 1985, she joined the faculty of the Johns Hopkins University School of Hygiene and Public Health and School of Medicine. During 1991–1992, she spent 6 months on sabbatical leave assisting the Vaccine Development Unit of WHO's Global Program on AIDS, helping to establish AIDS vaccine evaluation units in Uganda, Brazil, and Thailand. Dr. Clements is a member of several professional societies and serves on the Advisory Committee on Immunization Practices and the National Consultative Group for Vaccine Development.

Ciro de Quadros, M.D., M.P.H., is the Senior Adviser on Immunization for the Pan American Health Organization (PAHO). Since 1977 he has been responsible for the implementation of the Expanded Program on

Immunization (EPI) in the Region of the Americas, according to policies and strategies outlined by PAHO's directing bodies. He is also the Technical Secretary of the PAHO's Immunization Technical Advisory Group and of an Inter-Agency Coordinating Committee, which collaborates to enhance the implementation of EPI in the Americas, including the efforts to eradicate poliomyelitis. He is the editor of the PAHO publication "EPI Newsletter." Dr. de Quadros received his medical degree as well as his M.P.H in Brazil, the latest one in the National School of Public Health in Rio de Janeiro, where he served as Senior Lecturer in Epidemiology before joining the World Health Organization's Smallpox Eradication Program as the Chief Epidemiologist for the program in Ethiopia from 1970 to 1976. Dr. de Quadros is a member of the Task Force for Child Survival and Development and of several professional and scientific associations.

Michael A. Epstein, J.D., is a nationally recognized expert in intellectual property law, and a Partner in the international law firm Weil, Gotshal & Manges. He graduated from the New York University School of Law and Lehigh University (concentrating in biology and chemistry), both with high honors. His current practice involves both litigation and transactional work, including structuring and negotiating technology and intellectual property acquisitions, technology transfer and licensing arrangements, and joint ventures and other targeted alliances. He is the author of several books on intellectual property, including *Modern Intellectual Property, Drafting License Agreements,* and *International Intellectual Property,* as well as numerous articles on intellectual property law. Mr. Epstein has lectured frequently on intellectual property matters including trade secrets, biotechnology law, computer law, unfair competition, trademark law, and licensing agreements. He is a founder and co-editor of *The Journal of Proprietary Rights* and a member of the Editorial Board of the *Computer Lawyer.*

Ronald W. Hansen, Ph.D., is Associate Dean for Academic Affairs at the William E. Simon Graduate School of Business Administration. He came to the School in 1971 as Assistant Professor and became Director of the Systems Analysis Program in 1972. From 1977 to 1986, he was the Associate Director of the Center for Research in Government Policy and Business, now the Bradley Policy Research Center. He was the first recipient of the Merrell Dow Professorship of Pharmaceutical Administration in the College of Pharmacy at the Ohio State University (1986–1988). Dr. Hansen is widely recognized for his research in drug development policy and regulation of the pharmaceutical industry. He has presented papers in the United States, Sweden, Australia, Canada, and Switzerland. In addition, he helped establish, and is economic consultant to, the Center for the Study of Drug Development. Formerly a member of the National Advisory Council on Health Care Technology Assessment (1985–1988), Dr. Hansen has also been a consultant to the congressional Office of Technology Assessment for a panel on the Patent Term Restoration Act.

Donald E. Hill, B.S., retired from his position as Director of Product Certification, Center for Biologics Evaluation and Research, U.S. Food and Drug Administration (FDA), in 1990, and is now a Regulatory Consultant to the biologics industry. Mr. Hill received his B.S. degree from Ohio State University College of Pharmacy in 1960. In the same year, he received a commission into the U.S. Public Health Service, where he served his entire government career of 30 years. As Director of Product Certification, he was directly involved in the licensing and quality control of biological products in the United States. He provided guidance to industry on facility requirements, licensing standards, joint manufacturing arrangements, and product promotion and advertisement. Mr. Hill has published several articles on FDA facility and licensing requirements for manufacturers of biologics and is a frequent guest lecturer at industry and professional society meetings and at educational seminars. In 1987, he was honored with the R. E. Greco Award as Regulatory Professional of the Year.

John Lloyd Huck, B.S., retired from his position as Chairman of the Board of Merck and Co., Inc., in 1986. After receiving his B.S. degree in chemistry from Pennsylvania State University, he served in the U.S. Army Air Corps during World War II. Mr. Huck began his career in the pharmaceutical industry as a research chemist with Hoffmann LaRoche in 1946. In 1958, Mr. Huck joined the Merck Sharp & Dohme Division of Merck & Co., Inc., as Director of Marketing. After progressing through a number of marketing and managerial positions, he was elected President and Chief Operating Officer of Merck & Co., Inc., in 1978 and Chairman of the Board in 1985. After retiring from Merck in 1986, he joined the Board of Directors of Nova Pharmaceutical Corporation and served as Chairman of the Board and Chief Executive Officer for several years. He is past Chairman of the Board of Pennsylvania State University and of the Morristown Memorial Hospital. In addition, he has served on the boards of a number of corporate, professional, and not-for-profit organizations.

David T. Karzon, M.D., is Professor in the Departments of Pediatrics and Microbiology and Immunology, Vanderbilt University School of Medicine. He received a B.S. and M.S. from Ohio State University and his M.D. from the Johns Hopkins University School of Medicine. Dr. Karzon has taught since 1948, including 16 years at the State University of New York at Buffalo in both the Department of Bacteriology and Immunology and the Department of Pediatrics. Concurrently, he held an appointment as Director of the New York State Virology Laboratory, Buffalo, New York. From 1968 to 1986, Dr. Karzon served as Pediatrician-in-Chief, Vanderbilt University Hospital, Chair of the Department of Pediatrics, and Medical Director of the Children's Hospital of the Vanderbilt University Medical Center. He is currently Professor of Pediatrics as well as Professor of Microbiology and Immunology at Vanderbilt University Medical Center. Dr. Karzon has received awards from the U.S. Public Health Service, the Lowell M. Palmer Senior Fellowship, the Markle Scholar in Medical Science, and the Research Career Awards, U.S. Public Health Service, National Institutes of Health. He has served on several advisory committees and currently sits on the National Vaccine Advisory Committee.

Thomas D. Kiley, J.D., is an attorney, investor, and consultant residing in Hillsborough, California. He received his B.S. in chemical engineering from Pennsylvania State University and J.D. with highest distinction from the George Washington University School of Law. He is a member of the board of directors of Athena Neurosciences, Inc.; Cellpro, Inc.; GenPharm International, Inc.; InSite Vision, Inc.; Pharmacyclics, Inc.; Signition, Inc.; Geron Corporation; and the Argent Biosciences Fund. Mr. Kiley served as an Examiner at the U.S. Patent and Trademark Office from 1965 to 1967 and as Patent Solicitor for E. I. du Pont de Nemours & Co., Inc., from 1967 to 1969. From 1969 to 1980, Mr. Kiley practiced with the Los Angeles law firm of Lyon & Lyon, specializing in patent and other intellectual property litigation. From 1980 to 1988, he was an officer of Genentech, Inc., serving variously as Vice President and General Counsel, Vice President for Legal Affairs, and Vice President for Corporate Development.

Richard T. Mahoney, Ph.D., is Vice President and Director of Technology Promotion at the Program for Appropriate Technology in Health (PATH). He received a B.A. from Purdue University and his Ph.D. from the University of California, San Diego. Before joining PATH, Dr. Mahoney worked for the Ford Foundation's Population Office, where he was responsible for the international program in scientific research and development of fertility control. In 1979, he began as a representative for PATH in Asia, serving in Manila and Jakarta for 4 years. His current responsibilities at PATH include management of licensing, patents, copyrights, and trademarks; financing of business ventures; and the formulation of product development strategies and feasibility studies. Dr. Mahoney is a Founding Member of the International Task Force for

Hepatitis B Immunization and has written over 20 publications in chemistry, family planning, and vaccine-related topics.

Wendy K. Mariner, J.D., LL.M., M.P.H., presently holds three academic appointments: Professor, Boston University School of Public Health; Professor of Socio-Medical Science and Community Medicine, Boston University School of Medicine; and Lecturer in Social Medicine, Harvard Medical School. She is also a senior faculty member of the Law, Medicine and Ethics Program at Boston University. Ms. Mariner received her B.A. from Wellesley College, J.D. from Columbia University Law School, LL.M. from New York University Law School, and M.P.H. from the Harvard School of Public Health. She has lectured and published on such topics as drug and vaccine policy, patient's rights, and health care reform.   The research grants that she has received include Legal and Ethical Issues in AIDS Vaccine Development, Comparison of Compensation Programs for Vaccine Injury, and Informed Consent in Childhood Immunization. She is contributing editor to *Health Law and Ethics* for the American Journal of Public Health, and serves as a member of the AIDS Policy Advisory Committee at the National Institutes of Health.

David C. Mowery, Ph.D., is Associate Professor of Business and Public Policy at the Walter A. Haas School of Business, University of California at Berkeley. He received his undergraduate and doctoral degrees in economics from Stanford University, was a postdoctoral research fellow at the Harvard Business School, and has taught at Carnegie-Mellon University.   His research deals with the economics of technological innovation and the impact of public policy on innovation. During 1987 to 1988, Dr. Mowery served as Study Director for the National Academy of Sciences' Panel on Technology and Employment. In 1988, he served in the Office of the U.S. Trade Representative as a Fellow for the Council on Foreign Relations, International Affairs. He has testified before congressional committees, been a consultant for various federal agencies and industrial firms, and has written and edited several books. These include *Technology and the Pursuit of Economic Growth, Alliance Politics and Economics: Multinational Joint Ventures in Commercial Aircraft, Technology and Employment: Innovation and Growth in the U.S. Economy, The Impact of Technology Change on Employment and Economic Growth*, and *International Collaborative Ventures in U.S. Manufacturing.*

Mark Novitch, M.D., is Vice Chair of the Board of the Upjohn Company. He is responsible for pharmaceutical control, regulatory affairs, strategy and planning, business development, legal and government affairs, and public relations. He received a B.A. from Yale University and M.D. from New York Medical College. His medical staff positions and experience include Peter Bent Brigham Hospital and Harvard Medical School. He also worked as Assistant to the Deputy Assistant Secretary for Health and Scientific Affairs and was Assistant Staff Director of the Task Force on Prescription Drugs from 1967 to 1969. In addition, Dr. Novitch served as Federal Executive Fellow at the Brookings Institution from 1970 to 1971. Subsequently, after serving as Deputy Commissioner of the U.S. Food and Drug Administration (FDA), he went on to become Acting Commissioner of the FDA from 1983 to 1984. Dr. Novitch serves as President of the United States Pharmaceutical Convention. In addition, he serves on the Board of Directors of the American Foundation for Pharmaceutical Education, the National Fund for Medical Education, and the Council on Excellence in Government and is a Trustee of Kalamazoo College.

Suryanarayan Ramachandran, Ph.D., is the immediate Past Secretary of the Department of Biotechnology, Government of India. He obtained his master's degree from Banaras Hindu University, India, and his Ph.D. from the University of Illinois. For many years, he worked in the area of microbial biochemistry. As a visiting scientist at the Indiana University Medical Center (1967–1968), he worked on insulin antibodies and diabetic ketoacidosis. As Head of the Biochemistry Department of the Hindustan Antibiotics Research Center, and later as its Research Director, he was associated with characterization and the modes of action of antibiotics. He and his colleagues did extensive work on enzymes of both medical and industrial importance. He has several publications in these areas, as well as patents on large-scale immobilization of enzymes and enzyme-linked immunosorbent assay-based immunodiagnostic kits. From 1978 to 1982 he was the Chief Executive of Bengal Immunity Ltd., Calcutta, where he piloted the development of improved technologies for antimalarial agent production and the development of new technologies for antibacterial vaccines and antitoxins. In 1982, he was appointed the first member Secretary of the Interministerial National Biotechnology Board formed by the Government of India, and in 1986, he was appointed Secretary of the Department of Biotechnology. In this position, he guided the initiation of a number of programs in modern biology and biotechnology. He is a member of the Biotechnology Advisory Committee of the United Nations Educational, Scientific, and Cultural Organization; chair, Management Advisory Committee, Children's Vaccine Initiative; and a member of the Working Party of the United Nations Conference on Sustainable Development. He is an elected fellow of the National Academy of Medical Sciences, India; and the National Academy of Sciences, India.

Anthony Robbins, M.D., M.P.A., is currently Professor of Public Health at the Boston University School of Medicine. Dr. Robbins received his B.A. from Harvard University, his M.D. from Yale University School of Medicine, and his M.P.A. from John F. Kennedy School of Government, Harvard University. From 1981 to 1986, he served as a staff member for the Committee on Energy and Commerce, U.S. House of Representatives. Other past positions include Director, National Institute for Occupational Safety and Health, U.S. Department of Health and Human Services; Executive Director, Colorado Department of Health; and State Health Commissioner, Vermont Department of Health. Other academic institutions with which Dr. Robbins has been affiliated include McGill University and the Harvard Medical School and School of Public Health. He also served as President of the American Public Health Association in 1983 and has published several articles on vaccine development, supply, and policy over the last several years.

Jerald C. Sadoff, M.D., Colonel (MC), U.S. Army, is currently the Director of the Division of Communicable Diseases and Immunology, Walter Reed Army Institute of Research (WRAIR), where he is responsible for directing the Department of Defense's development, production and testing of vaccines against shigella, cholera, enterotoxigenic *Escherichia coli*, typhoid, *Neisseria meningitidis*, *Neisseria gonorrhoeae*, pseudomonas, lipid A, hepatitis A and E viruses, dengue, malaria, and leishmania. He serves as chairman of the Program for Vaccine Development Committee on Diarrheal Diseases of the United Nations Development Program/World Health Organization (UNDP/WHO) and as Chairman of the UNDP/WHO Program for Vaccine Development (PVD), Task Force in Oral Delivery of Vaccines; and Chairman of the UNDP/WHO PVD Task Force on Cholera. He is also a member of the UNDP/WHO PVD Committee on Trans-Disease Vaccinology. He has been an attending physician in Internal Medicine and Infectious Diseases at Walter Reed Hospital since 1972. He received his B.A. and M.D. from the University of Minnesota and completed internal medicine and infectious diseases graduate training at the Minneapolis Veterans Hospital. He was an Infectious Disease Officer in the Department of Bacterial Diseases from 1972, where he became chief in 1987. He is an Associate Professor of Medicine of the Uniformed Services University of the Health Sciences. Dr. Sadoff is a member of several scientific societies, including the Infectious Disease Society of America, the American Society for Microbiology, the American Venereal Disease Association, the Pseudomonas Club (Founding Member), and the International Endotoxin Society. He has received the Paul A. Siple Memorial Medallion, the Impact Meritorious Service Medal, and the Legion of Military Medical Merit.

Jay Philip Sanford, M.D., is Professor of Medicine, University of Texas Southwestern Medical School, and Dean Emeritus, Uniformed Services University of the Health Sciences (USUHS). He received his M.D. with honors from the University of Michigan Medical School in 1952 and Doctor of Military Medicine (honoris causa) from USUHS in 1991. Dr. Sanford served as Dean of the School of Medicine of USUHS beginning in 1975, became President of the University in 1981, and retired in 1991. In 1992, he was reappointed Professor of Medicine at the University of Texas Southwestern Medical School. Other past professional positions that Dr. Sanford has held include Chief, Bacteriology Laboratory, Parkland Memorial Hospital, Dallas, Texas, and Professor of Internal Medicine, University of Texas Southwestern Medical School. Dr. Sanford has received numerous honors, including the Distinguished Public Service Medal and the Distinguished Civilian Service Medal, U.S. Department of Defense; the Bristol Award, Infectious Disease Society of America; Medaille d'Honneur du Service de Sante des Armees (France); and Member, Institute of Medicine (IOM). In his professional career, Dr. Sanford has served on numerous advisory committees, boards, and panels, including several at the National Institutes of Health, the U.S. Food and Drug Administration, the National Aeronautics and Space Administration, the U.S. Department of Defense, the American Board of Internal Medicine, the Centers for Disease Control and Prevention, and the U.S. Public Health Service. These committee assignments included two terms on the Advisory Committee on Immunization Practices, the Armed Forces Epidemiologic Board Commission on Immunization, the Bureau of Biologics Panel on Review of Bacterial Vaccines and Toxoids, the IOM Committee on Private-Public Sector Relations in Vaccine Development (Chairman), and the IOM Board on Health Promotion-Disease Prevention. He is author of 190 articles in peer-reviewed journals and 130 textbook chapters.

George R. Siber, M.D., is the Director of the Massachusetts Public Health Biologic Laboratories, a state-operated and federally licensed facility that produces vaccines against diptheria, tetanus, and pertussis and other diseases for Massachusetts. He received his B.Sc. from Bishop's University, Quebec, and his M.D. from McGill University. He has been an Associate Professor of Medicine at Harvard Medical School since 1986 and has served as Attending Physician for Infectious Diseases Services at Beth Israel Hospital, Dana-Farber Cancer Institute, The Children's Hospital, and Brigham and Women's Hospital. His primary research interests have been in the development of vaccines and immune globulins directed against specific infections and in the assessment of the human immune response to vaccines. He is a member of the American College of Physicians, the American

Society for Microbiology, the Infectious Diseases Society of America, the Pediatric Infectious Disease Society, the International Endotoxin Society, and the Society for Pediatric Research.

Jane E. Sisk, Ph.D., Professor in the Division of Health Policy and Management, joined the faculty at the Columbia University School of Public Health in January 1992. She holds a Ph.D. in economics from McGill University, an M.A. in economics from George Washington University, and a B.A. with honors in international relations from Brown University. From 1981 to 1992 she directed health policy projects at the Congressional Office of Technology Assessment, where she was a Senior Associate and Project Director in the Health Program. Her reports addressed such topics as information for consumers on the quality of medical care, Medicare payment for physician services, Medicare payment for recombinant erythropoietin, federal policies toward the medical devices industry, and the cost-effectiveness of influenza and pneumococcal vaccines. Dr. Sisk is the immediate past President of the International Society of Technology Assessment in Health Care. Her research interests include technology assessment, prevention, and the organization and financing of medical care.

STAFF

Violaine S. Mitchell, MSc., is a Program Officer in the Division of International Health of the Institute of Medicine (IOM). She received her B.A. in development studies from Brown University and her MSc. in tropical public health from the Harvard School of Public Health. Prior to joining the IOM in 1990, she spent several years in Egypt running an animal health and production project among Cairo's traditional garbage collectors, the *zabbaleen.* Other projects during her three years at the National Academy of Sciences and the Institute of Medicine include work with the Committee on Malaria Prevention and Control, Board on International Health, and the International Forum for AIDS Research. Ms. Mitchell is a recipient of the Institute of Medicine 1991 Staff Achievement Award for her work on the Institute of Medicine report *Malaria: Obstacles and Opportunities* (1991).

Nalini Philipose joined the Division of International Health in October 1991 to work as a Research Assistant for the study on the Children's Vaccine Initiative. She graduated in May 1991 from Cornell University with a B.A. in Soviet Studies and Political Science. She was actively involved in all aspects of the study, from the formation of the committee to writing chapters of the report. She will attend Stanford Law School this fall.

Delores H. Sutton has an Associate Degree in Business Administration from the University of the District of Columbia and the University of Maryland. She joined the Institute of Medicine in 1987 and served as Assistant to the Director, Division of Health Care Services, until September 1992. She provides support for the Children's Vaccine Initiative Study, the Study on Female Morbidity and Mortality in Sub-Saharan Africa, and the Board on International Health. She is responsible for the logistics of meetings, travel and hotel arrangements for committees and staff, briefing materials, study files, correspondence, memos for staff, and assists with projects outside the immediate office.

Greg W. Pearson is a self-employed writer and editor with an expertise in the sciences, science policy, and health. He received a B.A. (1981) in biology from Swarthmore College and a master's in journalism (1988) from The American University. Over the past 4 years, Greg has worked on a number of projects for the Institute of Medicine and the National Academy of Sciences. He served as a consultant for the Children's Vaccine Study, Institute of Medicine.

Robert D. Crangle is an attorney and has been president of the Rose & Crangle, Ltd. management consulting firm since 1984. He received his Management Consultant certificate in 1980 from the Institute of Management Consultants and his J.D. from Harvard Law School in 1969. Mr. Crangle also received a B.S. from Kansas State University in 1966. His expertise is in human resources, science policy, government operations, information systems, economic development, and juridical services. He served as a consultant for the Children's Vaccine Initiative Study.

K

Acronyms

AAP	American Academy of Pediatrics
ACIP	Advisory Committee on Immunization Practices
AID	U.S. Agency for International Development
ANDA	abbreviated new drug application
BCG	bacillus Calmette-Guérin (vaccine against tuberculosis)
CBER	Center for Biologics Evaluation and Research (U.S. Food and Drug Administration)
CDC	Centers for Disease Control and Prevention
CDF	Children's Defense Fund
CPI	Consumer Price Index
CRADA	Cooperative Research and Development Agreement
CVI	Children's Vaccine Initiative
DOD	U.S. Department of Defense
DTP	diphtheria and tetanus toxoids and pertussis vaccine
ELA	Establishment License Application
EPI	Expanded Program on Immunization (World Health Organization)
FDA	U.S. Food and Drug Administration
FTEs	full-time equivalents
GLPs	Good Laboratory Practices
GMPs	Good Manufacturing Practices
Hib-CV	*Haemophilus influenzae* type b vaccine, conjugated
HIV	human immunodeficiency virus
ICIDR	International Collaborations in Infectious Disease Research

IND	Investigational New Drug
IOM	Institute of Medicine
MMR	measles, mumps, and rubella vaccine
MOD	March of Dimes Birth Defects Foundation
NAV	North American Vaccine
NIAID	National Institute of Allergy and Infectious Diseases
NICHD	National Institute of Child Health and Human Development
NIH	National Institutes of Health
NVA	National Vaccine Authority
NVAC	National Vaccine Advisory Committee
NVICP	National Vaccine Injury Compensation Program
NVP	National Vaccine Program
OPV	oral polio vaccine
PAHO	Pan American Health Organization
PLA	Product License Application
PPPI	Pharmaceutical Producer Price Index
PTO	Patent and Trademark Office
PVD	Program for Vaccine Development (United Nations Development Program/World Health Organization)
R&D	research and development
RIVM	Rijksinstituut voor Volgezondheid en Milieuhygiene (National Institute of Public Health and Environmental Protection, The Netherlands)
SB	SmithKline Beecham
TT	tetanus toxoid
UNDP	United Nations Development Program
UNICEF	United Nations Children's Fund
USAMMDA	U.S. Army Medical Material Development Activity
USAMRIID	U.S. Army Medical Research Institute of Infectious Diseases
VAERS	Vaccine Adverse Events Reporting System
WHO	World Health Organization